PENGUIN BOOKS

Care of the Dying

Richard Lamerton was born in Yorkshire and educated at Bradford Grammar School and St Barth-
olomew's Hospital, London. He was Medical Officer
at St Joseph's Hospice in Hackney, and then became
a Clinical Assistant at St Christopher's Hospice,
Sydenham, which he combined with general practice.
For a three-year term Dr Lamerton was Chairman of
the Human Rights Society. From 1979 until 1982 he
was Medical Director of the Macmillan Service, a
home care service for dying patients and their families
in the East End of London. He is married and has
two daughters.

Richard Lamerton

Care of the Dying

Revised and Expanded Edition

PENGUIN BOOKS

PENGUIN BOOKS

Published by the Penguin Group
Penguin Books Ltd, 27 Wrights Lane, London W8 5TZ, England
Viking Penguin, a division of Penguin Books USA Inc,
375 Hudson Street, New York, New York 10014, USA
Penguin Books Australia Ltd, Ringwood, Victoria, Australia
Penguin Books Canada Ltd, 2801 John Street, Markham, Ontario, Canada L3R 1B4
Penguin Books (NZ) Ltd, 182–190 Wairau Road, Auckland 10, New Zealand

Penguin Books Ltd, Registered Offices: Harmondsworth, Middlesex, England

First published by Priory Press Limited 1973
Revised and expanded edition published in Pelican Books 1980
Reprinted in Penguin Books 1990
1 3 5 7 9 10 8 6 4 2

Printed and bound in Great Britain by
Cox & Wyman Ltd, Reading
Set in Linotype Baskerville

Contents

Introduction

A leader in the *Lancet* of 3 June 1978 declared that 'Soon incompetence in terminal care will be recognized for what it is.'[210]* This books seeks to advance that day. As well as sharing our experience of hospice care for dying people with our colleagues in the caring professions, it is also hoped that public demand for good terminal care will be stimulated. If people's expectations of better care are raised, then medical and nursing training will have to meet the higher standard.

There is undoubtedly room for improvement among the professions; but to be fair, care of the dying can give rise to difficult situations which quite reasonably perplex most of us. For example, how many doctors could tell you that the commonest cause of vomiting in a patient with widespread cancer is constipation, and that vomiting is not the rule even in patients with advanced cancer of the stomach, provided that their bowels are empty? And although district nurses are supposed to pay bereavement visits to families, how many actually do? Or how many, when they get there, wish they knew how to handle the situation, and how to tell normal grief from pathological danger-signs?

How do you cope with the family which insists that a dying patient must not be told what is wrong with him, even when you suspect that he knows already and needs a thorough discussion and reassurance?

We have found that it takes a doctor or nurse at least a year to be really proficient and confident in such situa-

* Please see pp. 213–33 for numbered references.

tions, even when working with dying patients all the time. Would it not help to have available someone who had made a special study of care of the dying? I am, in fact, saying that while everyone could do better, our dying patients would be best served if specialists in their care were trained and available throughout the health services.

No doubt the suggestion makes many professionals puff out their feathers and say they need no help. Midwives met the same sort of resistance, but have managed to convince the world that, while any old nurse can deliver a baby, most women nowadays would prefer to have a specialist around. Just so, while most of us could succeed in dying somehow or other even with no help, it would be a great comfort to know that one would be attended by someone confident, knowledgeable and experienced in modern techniques of care of the dying.

Happily a cadre of specially trained nurses, doctors and social workers is beginning to emerge in Britain. This welcome development means that we can now ask whether health authorities are really meeting their obligations to the patient if they do not, for example, have one of their nurses trained in this way on the district, and one in each general hospital?

As this book aims to show, such people could make a great difference to the dignity and comfort of the average man at the end of his life.

This Penguin edition draws heavily on articles I have written in *Nursing Times* and *World Medicine*. I wish to thank the editors for permission to use this material. I would like to thank the patients and staff of the Macmillan Service, St Joseph's Hospice in Hackney and St Christopher's Hospice in Sydenham for giving me so much help in preparing this book, and for being a constant inspiration and support. In typing the manuscript Miss P. Davison and Mrs C. Kheir-Eldin showed the combined qualities of a gladiator and Robert the Bruce's spider. My thanks to them, and also to the National Society for Cancer Relief who paid them. Without this charity giving its massive support, care of the dying as a body of special knowledge would have taken much longer to develop – indeed might have foundered completely.

Inevitably most of the patients whose care is described in this book have cancer. It is concerned with people who have a progressive, inevitably fatal condition and whose prognosis of life is probably only a few months or weeks. Geriatric care – for instance of people with heart disease or strokes – and the care of younger people with such conditions as multiple sclerosis are not within the scope of this study. Patients with widespread cancer, however, usually are, though the science of oncology is already having considerable success in the control or even cure of some kinds of cancer.

1. The Needs

It is never true that 'nothing more can be done' for a patient. It may be useless to continue treatment with curative drugs or surgery, but one can still give attention and friendship, relief and comfort.[65] Sometimes a dying patient in hospital is looked on by the staff as one of their failures, while if he is at home, the nursing may prove too heavy for his family.

When a man is dying, active treatment of disease becomes increasingly irrelevant to his real needs. In the case of progressive incurable illness, the last three months of life are generally regarded as the period called 'dying'. It is, however, difficult to assess with any accuracy the duration of life left to a man.[283]

With good care, a patient can die without distress. Techniques are available whereby pain can be relieved, as can most of the other unpleasant symptoms which we commonly associate with dying. Nausea, for instance, and breathlessness can at least be eased until they are no longer in the forefront of the patient's attention. If there is physical distress as death approaches, it is probably because these newly-developed techniques which could bring relief are not being used.[339]

When we are called to advise on the further management of patients with widespread cancer – often in a hospital ward – we find the same picture of needless misery with frustrating repetitiveness. It is usually characterized by inadequate pain control, blocked bowels due to impacted motions, bedsores, and thrush in the mouth.

And if this physical suffering is bad, the emotional isolation is even worse. So often the patient is told lies about his diagnosis and the family are advised that he should never know the truth. Communication with him thus ceases, compounded in hospital by his being hidden in a side room, omitted from the consultant's ward round, and sedated.[162] I commonly meet the patient who is begging for information about his diagnosis or life-expectancy, who does not believe the bland reassurances given him, who has seen his wife retreat hastily with tears in her eyes, and is indignant that no one will treat him like a responsible adult.[303] Worse than that, how often do I meet the terrified patient, fearing some awful but in fact highly unlikely fate like bursting or choking or screaming in agony, who cannot be reassured because no one will let him talk. It is widely assumed by laymen that death from cancer must be violent. In fact this is almost never the case. If communication is allowed to flow, reassurance and a promise of help can eliminate so much fear.

These fears are the fuel with which the euthanasia lobby stokes its sinister fire.[67] Its existence is an indictment of present-day care of the dying.[26]

The Need for Teaching

Terminal care involves a complete change of priorities for doctors and nurses. Their aim is now no longer to cure the patient; instead they work to keep him comfortable and both the medical and emotional needs of the patient have to be met effectively.[334]

Nurses and medical students all over the world need teaching in this field.[15] The student who stands tongue-tied before a dying man realizes how little he understands the patient's needs or how to cope with them. He will probably learn most from an inter-disciplinary discussion group, for in their care of the dying the doctor, priest and nurse have much to learn from each other.[164]

But in even straightforward practical matters teaching

is inadequate. Nearly every nurse I meet knows perfectly well, from experience, that pain-killing drugs like pethidine and pentazocine (also called Fortral) have a duration of action of only about two hours. Yet the doctors are not told.[242] Taught in medical school that these drugs have a duration of four hours, doctors prescribe them as such and then go away. Only the nurse is around to see the pain return.

All nurses should be shown cases of thrush in the mouth and taught to recognize it. They should also be taught how to diagnose and treat constipation. Care of mouths and bowels is surely part of basic nursing, yet it is bowel care which is the most sadly neglected. Exactly 9% of the last 1,000 patients referred to our care had a bowel impaction which had to be unblocked by hand. Patients referred to us by district nurses generally fared slightly better – it is the patients surrounded all day by health care professionals in a hospital who are the most likely to die of constipation.[202]

In a survey of *Life Before Death* (Cartwright, 1973 – see Bibliography) it was found that as few as 2% of patients in a teaching hospital may be there for terminal care. But 22% of the patients in the beds of a district general hospital will die, in those beds, within a year. So unless teaching hospitals deliberately incorporate teaching on care of the dying into their curricula, it can be easily overlooked, and the newly-qualified doctor can find himself alarmingly unprepared for the demands of his first job.[49]

The Need for Research

Although it is now possible to relieve much of the suffering of the dying, many unanswered questions still remain. More research is urgently needed.[37] It took some years to break the back of pain, and there is still room for improvement. Other symptoms need further carefully controlled trials, and the field of psychotherapy – both for the dying and for the bereaved – is being explored. We do not yet know enough about the process of normal healthy death, let alone about its pathology.

At community level, there is a need for more teaching of and research into the care of the dying, so that one day we may all say with Francis Bacon,

'It is as natural to die as to be born.'[18]

The Need for Hospices

Many people die peacefully in their sleep, requiring little or no medical attention. Over 60% of the British population die in hospital. In New York State the figure has passed 72%. Those who die quickly from such causes as accidents, strokes, suicide or heart attacks do not involve the hospital staff in any change of priorities, and can be cared for in the everyday working. The elderly who die gently in the embrace of the 'Old Man's Friend' (pneumonia – see p. 124), can usually be cared for at home by the family doctor and his team – again with no difficulty. But there will always be those who, like King Charles,[225] are 'an unconscionable time a-dying', and whose demise is likely to be attended by distress.

For instance, one in five of us will die of cancer. Special care will be needed if the cancer proves painful (which in about 40% of patients it does not).[169] Other people who may need specialized terminal care are some of those with certain neurological disease – such as motor neurone disease[302] (amyotrophic lateral sclerosis) or Huntington's chorea – which may, if they progress severely enough, lead to the death of the patient. Other smaller groups needing this care would include a few of the people suffering from kidney, heart or liver failure, or brain injuries from accidents. Most of my observations have been made with the larger group, the cancer patients, though of course a diagnosis of cancer does not necessarily mean a death warrant: all manner of cures are now possible.

This period of terminal illness is very wearying for the

patients, both physically and mentally, and is often a time when they receive much less medical and social support than they require.[316] Cottage hospitals, staffed by local family doctors, may sometimes be an enormous help,[310] particularly in country districts. To fill this gap in health care in towns, however, institutions called hospices have come into being. The patient who does not need the manifold and costly resources of a general hospital and who cannot be at home is frequently better cared for, and happier, in a smaller specialized unit.[71]

Surveys in the sixties which gave impetus to the launching of the hospice movement revealed much suffering and anguish.[111] One fifth of dying patients in hospitals were in severe unrelieved pain. Two thirds of cancer patients being looked after at home had severe or moderate suffering,[230] and this was only improved to 44% by a GP who was aware of the problem and bothered to assess it.[312] Clearly, if people are to die at home in a state that is at all civilized, extra help of a specialist nature is going to be needed.[216]

But a general hospital is not the best place for a patient in need of special terminal care. So often he finds himself either hidden in a lonely side room or else exposed to a ward of thirty or more patients who are having surgical operations or making tantalizing recoveries while he goes downhill.

It is difficult, in a busy ward, with all its demands on the staff, to give a dying patient the understanding of his problems and the discriminating handling of the drugs that he needs to ease his symptoms. Inevitably much distress which could be relieved has to be overlooked.[259] What is needed is a team of doctors and nurses with time just to sit and listen: time to sort out symptoms and any other personal problems, time to help the patient to understand and adjust to his situation at his own pace. This applies equally to other members of the staff. There must be sensitive communication among the whole caring team – doctor, nurse, social worker, chaplain, physiotherapist and so on – so that as the patient's insight into his condition increases, his progress may be fully known to everyone who approaches him. Such a close-knit team is less likely to arise in a general hospital than in a small establishment like a hospice. A 'terminal ward' tacked on to a big hospital would also have its disadvantages: other staff in the hospital would not always have the enlightened attitude to the dying which would be developed by those working in the unit, and if there were staff shortages, acute wards would naturally take precedence. For the patient the move would have the same significance as would a move to a hospice.

Since it is in the hospices that the methods of good care of the dying were first elucidated, I shall begin by examining their functioning. Then in subsequent chapters I will consider how their methods can be more widely disseminated in health services generally, and what are the philosophical implications of the new standard they set.

2. The Hospice Movement

The aim of Care of the Dying is to make the patient's body a comfortable enough place to live in so that he is free, if he wishes, to prepare for death mentally and spiritually.

It was this work which brought forth the present-day hospice movement, but the idea is much bigger. Deep in our common mind and heart, as old as our civilization itself, is the knowledge that hospitality is a duty owed to the weary traveller and to the sick. The modern hospital is often not a place of hospitality, yet that is its origin. The cold noisiness, the illusion of efficiency, the uninvolved staff fascinated by my liver function but not by me,[253] or quarrelling about their pay and holidays while waiting lists lengthen[344] – how did hospital get so far from hospitality?[73]

Throughout our history the love of giving and caring, of protecting the needy, has emerged again and again and its principles have been restated. 'Thou shalt love thy neighbour as thyself' (Matt. 19:19) re-echoes, sooner or later, in every sphere of human activity. It is the basis of our law of tort, the ecumenical factor in our religion, and the reason for medicine. In the eleventh century we hear the Knights Hospitalers of the Order of St John of Jerusalem in their hospices addressing their patients as 'Our Lords the Sick'. In 1476 Ficino found it necessary to say, 'The duty of a doctor when he visits the sick is to realize that a life is at stake, so that he dare not attempt anything without a reason nor without a purpose.' We hear Florence Nightingale saying, in 1859, 'It is quite surprising how many men practically behave as if the scientific end were the only one in view, or as if the sick body were but a reservoir for stowing medicines into, and the surgical disease only a curious case the sufferer has made for the attendant's special information.' And in our own century (1976) Dr Cicely Saunders wrote: 'What dying people need most of all is a doctor who will see them as another person: at very least, we can stand by them.'[336] Down through the ages it has been necessary to introduce correctives into the practice of medicine to prevent it becoming an entertainment (or, in modern jargon, 'employment') for those whose duty is the serious work of caring. The Hospice Movement of our day is just such a corrective, but it is based on long traditions and deep roots.

The word 'hospice' is reminiscent of the Middle Ages, when hundreds of hospices were dotted all over Europe, where travellers found food, refuge and spiritual encouragement to fit them for the journey ahead.

In the middle of the nineteenth century a lady with the memorable name of Mary Aikenhead opened the first modern hospice, in Dublin. She had founded an order of nuns, the Irish Sisters of Charity, and one of the tasks she set them was to care for people who were dying.

It was not long before the Sisters had many tales of woe about families coping with awful problems under conditions of poverty, ignorance and overcrowding. Mary Aikenhead therefore decided that a special kind of nursing home was needed for these patients, a home that was quieter and smaller than an acute hospital, but which had the same facilities for bedside nursing.

This great lady gave her own house in Dublin to be the first nursing home of this kind, and it was she who applied to it the old name 'hospice'. Since she considered death to be the beginning of a journey, a thoroughfare and not a terminus, the old name of the resting places on the pilgrimage to the Holy Land seemed the most appropriate.

The dawn of the twentieth century saw her Sisters opening another similar house in London (St Joseph's Hospice) along with two others started by Anglican nuns and one by the Methodist West London Mission.

This latter was St Luke's House for the Dying Poor, now called Hereford Lodge, and in 1894 its founder, Dr Howard Barrett, wrote:

> Many persons, when I tell them about St Luke's, say: 'What a very, very sad place! Don't you feel painfully depressed whenever you go there?'
> 'Not a bit,' I reply cheerfully, 'I find it delightful and invigorating.'
> And indeed I do. I know that there are hundreds and hundreds more up and down the dreary streets and courts of London, in just the same plight as those we have here ... to whom, while life shall last, we can give peace and rest, and much ease from pain, the best food, the best medicine, gentle hands to tend them, friendly voices to cheer them, and the good tidings of the all-embracing Love and the Eternal Life. This ought to be enough to make anyone cheerful.[24]

While this development was proceeding in Europe, the needs had also been perceived in America, where a parallel development had occurred.

Living next door to Louisa Alcott of *Little Women* fame, in Concord, Massachusetts, was the family of millionaire Nathaniel Hawthorne. His daughter Rose watched her friend Emma Lazarus (the poetess whose words are inscribed at the base of the Statue of Liberty) die of cancer, and began to wonder how the poor fared when similarly afflicted. She founded an order of Dominican nuns who devoted themselves to terminal care. Their first hospice opened in New York City in 1899. With later expansion of the order – the Servants of Relief for incurable cancer – six more homes opened elsewhere in the USA. In the 1950s a group of New York social workers started 'Cancer Care Inc.' to try to give support to people dying at home.

The hospice idea still awaited its full flowering, however. Two developments in the 1950s provided the necessary impetus. The first was the establishment of the Marie

Curie Foundation, which set out to fight the consequences of malignant disease. One of the needs which the Foundation's initial survey revealed was for more hospices.

'It is obvious to us,' said the report,

that considerable hardship exists in the case of many families who are taking care of one member with cancer at home. In addition to providing skilled nursing treatment for the patient, the provision of residential homes would save much mental suffering, stress and strain for the relatives. Beds in the hospitals might also be freed. We found that some old patients were very reluctant to leave their homes, even though conditions were often deplorable. It is possible that they would be prepared to enter a residential home rather than a public institution.[230]

The second great development in the fifties started through David Tasma, a Polish refugee from the Warsaw ghetto who died in 1948 in a London teaching hospital. He discussed his needs with the social worker, and between them they conceived of a special kind of care, in a home designed for the purpose. Certainly the medical expertise would be needed, but it would need to be appropriate care, given in an atmosphere of loving attention. 'I need what is in your mind and in your heart,' Mr Tasma told the social worker, and he gave her a gift of £500 'to be a window in your Home'. The social worker's name was Cicely Saunders. That commission involved her in a life's work. Already qualified as a nurse, she had to give up social work and study medicine. Having done so, she arrived at St Joseph's Hospice as its first full-time Medical Officer. She came to St Joseph's with a conviction that pain for the dying was unnecessary, and set about proving it.

From the development of her ideas a whole system of terminal care emerged. 'A unit for patients with advanced or terminal cancer,' she wrote,

does not have the challenge of diagnosis nor difficult decisions to make concerning radical treatment. It does not have the interest and encouragement of cure and only rarely of remission, but it is easier for its workers to look at their patients as people, to spend time with their relatives and to concentrate on the relief of distress whenever it appears. Above all it should be easier for them to give a patient the kind of unhurried attention he may need so greatly.

The staff in such a place have the fascination of knowing and watching each man come to terms with his illness in his own way and come along his own path to its ending. They have to learn to help people make this part of their lives into real living and not mere existing.[335]

Then followed years of work researching pain control, and developing the plans for this special kind of home and its care. Dr Saunders adopted Mary Aikenhead's title 'hospice', and St Christopher's was opened in July 1967.

The hospice idea 'embodies a rather rare combination of spirituality and hard medicine, a combination whose uniqueness may not be appreciated until one encounters it in such a person as Cicely Saunders.'[163]

In St Christopher's were drawn together all the threads of experience, from Europe and America, to be woven for the first time into a system of comprehensive care. Such a gathering of energy, like a deep intake of breath before the singing of a great aria, must be followed by a resounding explosion of revolutionary ideas. Now the secrets are out, and indeed widely acclaimed. The world has come to St Christopher's for its inspiration and encouragement. From all corners of the enlightened globe there now come stories of hospice groups being founded, struggling for funds, learning the techniques, broadcasting the news of better care.[171] In America, we hear Dennis Rezendes of the National Hospice Organization* now saying:

In the course of the next decade, the Hospice program will no longer be innovative, but will be folded right into the existing health-care system. Everybody in the health field will be sensitive to, and knowledgeable about, the care of terminally ill patients and their families.

*765 Prospect Street, New Haven, Connecticut 06511.

Indeed, following the lead of Dr Sylvia Lack in New Haven, who pioneered 'Hospice Inc.' – incorporated in 1971 – there has been a mushrooming of this kind of service in the USA.[447] Originally she worked in home care only, but in 1978 their hospice wards were built, to be opened in the following year. Hospice of Marin and San Diego Hospice and other California groups began home care services in the early seventies with a hospital Palliative Care Team in St Luke's Hospital, New York.[439] Then the American National Cancer Institute financed three hospice buildings – in Boonton, New Jersey; Tucson, Arizona;[139] and under the wing of the Kaiser Foundation in Los Angeles. Shortly after that the Veterans Administration involved itself in hospice development. Now there are over 400 groups in various stages of experience or planning all around the North American Continent.[8] They will have to be on their guard against involvement with euthanasia groups,[440] big business greed, cranky death-fascination cults and psychobabble enthusiasts who will not roll up their sleeves to *nurse* the patients.

In Europe we can see great interest in Britain, Ireland, Holland, Norway, Switzerland and several other countries. Each year brings news of many more developing teams. The British hospice movement is still the most advanced.[397] Its favoured pattern is to build a small unit in the grounds of a general hospital, using its facilities but administrationally independent of it. The National Society for Cancer Relief often builds these units, but they are then usually handed over to the National Health Service to run.[55] The dangers here are that bureaucrats may see an independent hospice as an erosion of their empire and want to manage it in the same way as they would a hospital. This could easily kill the spirit of a hospice, which is bound to be more akin to the spirit of a voluntary organization, running on devotion and much voluntary support. There is also the danger, on both sides of the Atlantic, of second-rate establishments riding on the bandwagon of the movement because they have been

around from its beginning and have not updated themselves in accord with the latest developments of the
seventies.

Of course one could hope that some day care of the
dying will be so good, and so thoroughly taught to
students, that hospices become obsolete because hospitals
and family doctors cope without trouble. But unless
special small units remain in every community to maintain the standards, I would be surprised if quite such a
revolution in attitudes occurred.

Sheila Hancock described the attitudes to her dying
mother, who was in a general hospital, and the distress
which she was caused, but then went on to speak about a
hospice's care for her husband:

> For me and my husband their method was 100% successful.
> It was a totally different experience from that with my mother.
>
> I understand that there is an increase in the numbers of
> people dying in hospitals. I would think that if home assistance
> could be better organized this would not be the case. I do think
> that people would prefer that those they loved died with
> them – I certainly did. I think they needed my comfort, they
> needed my love – which I could not expect a detached medical
> person to give. But you do need help; believe me you do need
> help.[140]

In a hospice setting the whole caring team can work
together and the doctors and nurses can develop the skills
the dying man needs. They can have time to listen when
needed and to help the whole family to come together
and say their farewells.[348]

Inevitably the team find themselves in a position to
teach others. A clear duty of any hospice is to set an
example from which other health care professionals can
learn. Hospices must be teaching units: nurses and social
workers, medical and theological students should have
opportunities to work in them for elective periods and
lecturing and training should be part of the everyday
work. Care of the dying can only really be learnt by
apprenticeship. Books and lectures could never replace

real experience at the bedside in the company of a master of the art. With whole groups of dying patients together there is also an opportunity for research into their needs and care.

But we must not lose sight of the original version of Mary Aikenhead. She saw her hospice as only a last resort if her Sisters could not cope with a patient at home. Most of us would prefer to die at home if at all possible, and this should be the aim of the health services.

A fully fledged hospice has a home care service which will cater for the needs of the dying and bereaved in the community by making its skills available to the family doctor. St Christopher's Hospice pioneered this return to Mary Aikenhead's original concept, and several others have since followed suit.[288] The result is that a hospice can nearly treble the number of patients under its care, catering for the needs of a whole city.

People often object that to reserve a small hospital entirely for the dying would earn it a macabre reputation in the locality and discourage doctors from referring patients. Some hospices have met this objection by having some long-stay patients alongside the dying ones so that it is not true that 'everyone in there is dying'.

But from experience of living near to two of the hospices, I can only say that a reputation for good care and a cheerful atmosphere travels much faster than a grim one. This is just not a problem if the hospice is working properly.[331]

It is also important to involve the local community in the unit so that it is familiar. Open days, a force of voluntary workers and social events all help in this integration. St Luke's in Sheffield runs a Day Hospital as part of the hospice service.[416]

For the patient himself, apprehension vaporizes in hours as his pain is banished, the light and cheerfulness of the place envelop him and he finds that people are really caring.

And what greater comfort could there be, as he comes

to realize that he is dying, than to see the man in the next bed die easily and peacefully? Several times patients have said to me, 'Well, if I can go like that, I don't mind going.'[218]

The application of the techniques of analytical diagnosis and scientific prescribing are as essential to a hospice as its quality of care. It will be making use of the whole field of medicine – palliative surgery[123] and radiotherapy, anti-tumour drugs and nerve blocks – to bring relief to its patients.

Our techniques must be good, but we must also give ourselves to the patients. It can be very lonely in hospital, and no amount of science will alleviate that. But one gentle cheerful nurse can. She need not be a Socrates – it is not the profundity of her understanding which is of value – but the fact that she cares enough to try. A nurse who was dying wrote about this as follows:

I know, you feel insecure, don't know what to say, don't know what to do. But please believe me, if you care, you can't go wrong. Just admit that you care. That is really for what we search. We may ask for whys and wherefores, but we don't really expect answers. Don't run away ... wait ... all I want to know is that there will be someone to hold my hand when I need it. I am afraid. Death may get to be a routine with you, but it is new to me. You may not see me as unique, but I've never died before, to me, once is pretty unique!

You whisper about my youth, but when one is dying, is he really so young any more? I have lots I wish we could talk about. It really would not take much of your time because you are in here quite a bit anyway.

If only we could be honest, both admit our fears, touch one another. If you really care, would you lose so much of your valuable professionalism if you even cried with me? Just person to person? Then, it might not be so hard to die ... in a hospital ... with friends close by.[14]

Essentials of a Hospice

It was TB which originally brought patients to the new hospices at the turn of this century. Then cancer took over, and the emphasis was changed. No doubt there will be other changes in the future, not only in the kind of patients cared for, not only in the range of medical specialties that are enhanced by this approach, but also in the way the principles are applied. In some communities the free-standing self-contained hospice[196] may be inappropriate. Cottage hospitals run by family doctors, departments of big hospitals – like the Palliative Care Unit in Montreal's Royal Victoria Hospital[125] – and teams based almost entirely on domiciliary care will no doubt find ways of implementing 'hospice care' appropriate to their time and place. Wars, social changes, technological revolutions may all make dinosaurs of our huge hospitals and many other of our institutions, but the simple caring embodied in the hospice movement will be needed wherever and whenever there is a human race.

For it is entirely clear by now that mere architecture, however pleasing, cannot make a hospice; and that true hospice care cannot be artificially programmed. Care is care. It is not a building, a grant, a law or a committee ... I hear of hospice committees now across the country studying other hospice committees, or calling in 'outside planners' – presumably to make elaborate and expensive outside plans of all that has not been happening inside. This is not hospice work; this is mere fiddling and politics. Hospice work does not begin with charts of administrative functions, or lists of potential sites, or willing benefactors. Hospice work begins with the question *What does this patient need?* – Sandol Stoddard (see Bibliography)

Returning to the word, and its origin, I would like to quote the research of Dr J. Morrison Hobson. In 1926[161] he published a study which traced 'hospice' and 'hospital' right back to their Sanskrit roots:

With the Romans, *hospes* stood both for a host and a guest. From a root *ghan* (Sanskrit हन् – han – to strike) came the

Latin *hasta*, a spear, *hostia* recompense, *hostis* an enemy or a foreigner and, strange as it may seem, the above word *hospes*. From this same common root were derived the English word *guest*, the Welsh *gwestai*, the Armoric *hostiz* and the Bohemian *host*, all having the same meaning, but also signifying a Stranger. How came it that applications apparently so diverse as 'host', 'guest' and 'stranger' each originated in the unamiable notion of striking a blow? Let us go back in imagination to primitive man. He is standing at the entrance to his cave or his hut. Presently a stranger approaches. 'Surely he is an enemy,' says he, 'where is my spear?' But as man advances towards civilization, we see him acting on the safer assumption that the stranger has no evil intent and resolved to disarm him morally, if so be he has such motive, by offering him food, or at least salt and shelter. Hence it became the customary duty of the man of the tent to give these to the wayfarer, asking no questions. From this conception it is not difficult to go further and understand how the Roman *hospes* signified both entertainer and entertained, *hospitalis* (hospitable) the quality which welcomed others, whether friends or strangers, and *hospitium* the place where guests were received. Hence the French acquired, in the one sense, the word *hospice*, where the helpless and the wayfarers were welcomed, as at Great St Bernard, established in the eleventh century for the accommodation of those traversing that dangerous pass in the Alps, and, in another, *hospital* (now *hôpital*) for the treatment of the sick. The English, probably borrowing from the Continent, applied from the beginning the word *inclusively* to places for the temporary reception of travellers and pilgrims and for the permanent care of the aged poor, the 'maimed, halt and blind', and for the cure of the sick. The monasteries also had their *hospitium* for guests or strangers, while their infirmary was not exclusively for their own sick.

In the twentieth century this hospitality is lavished in concrete ways. There is, for example, the pain control. 66% of the 607 patients admitted to St Christopher's Hospice in 1976–7 were referred with a pain problem. All but 10 patients ($\frac{1}{4}$%) obtained good relief from pain; and of those, four were in the hospice for less than 48 hours.[320]

This is the scientific ground on which the modern hospice movement is founded.

The combined experience of St Christopher's Hospice, London, and Hospice Inc., New Haven, led to the compiling of this list of essential features of hospice care:

1. *Management by an experienced clinical team* integrated into the work of the whole medical community and giving effective continuity of care.

2. *Understanding control of the common symptoms of terminal disease, especially pain in all its aspects,* will enable patients to live to their maximum potential and will at times herald unexpected remissions and/or the possibility of further active treatment.

3. *Skilled and experienced team nursing* which calls for confident leadership by the ward sister and easy communication among its members.

4. *A full inter-disciplinary staff* meeting frequently for discussion. The doctor does not relinquish his clinical responsibility but a member of another discipline may sometimes assume leadership for a particular patient or family.

5. *A Home Care Programme,* active or consultative and involving all the relevant disciplines, must be developed according to local circumstances so that it can be integrated with the hospitals, the family practices of the area and its own beds.

6. *Recognition of the patient and his family as the unit of care* and of the family as part of the caring team. They may need support, not only in meeting physical demands but also in their own search for reality and meaning.

7. *A mixed group of patients.* Although the current interest in hospice care in the US is especially concerned with 'the dying cancer patient and his family', a good community is usually a mixed one and hospices may include among their concerns those with long-term illness, chronic pain and, in some cases, frailty and old age.

8. *Bereavement follow-up* to identify those who are especially vulnerable and to give support in cooperation with the family doctor and any local services which can be involved.

9. *Methodical recording and analysis* will monitor clinical practice and, coordinated with relevant research where possible, lead to soundly based practice and teaching.

10. *Teaching in all aspects of terminal care.* Special units should be a resource, stimulating initial interest, giving experience and passing on tested knowledge to others in both general and specialist fields.

11. *Imaginative use of the architecture available.* Many hospices will not be able to build anew and have to adapt a building in order to combine privacy with openness and community and a sense of home with efficient operation.

12. *An efficient and approachable administration,* essential to any field of human need and care, is here required to give security to patients, families and staff. Efficiency is both comforting and time saving. So far, hospices have shown that their operation is cost effective as well as appropriate and humane.

13. *A readiness for the cost of commitment and the search for meaning.* Devotion has been an outstanding characteristic of past and present hospices. Willingness to face this demand has a fundamental bearing on the way the work is done and the stability of the staff. A Christian hospice will be aware of the presence of the crucified and risen Christ in the midst.[320]

When a new patient arrives at a hospice he is welcomed by name while still in the ambulance, and his future ward sister or staff nurse accompanies him to the ward. It is important that the relatives should also be welcomed, because henceforth treatment will be directed towards the whole family.[409] Suffering will not be confined to the patient himself: everyone who loves him will to some extent be a patient of the hospice.

Some aspects of nursing are intensified in caring for the

dying, and some fade into the background.[394] There arises, quite naturally, a certain reverence for the patients. This includes unresponsive patients, who must always be handled gently, and treated as if fully aware. Careless conversations over an apparently unconscious person are sometimes clearly heard by that person. It is usually considered that hearing is the last of the senses to fade, and many religions have accordingly provided special prayers to be read quietly into the ear of the dying man.

Routine procedures such as taking the temperature and pulse need not disturb the patient now as they are of no further practical use. On the other hand, attention to the patient's appearance is important in preserving his dignity. Even if there is no point in temperature-taking, the men should still be shaved regularly, and the ladies should have their hair done.

When his pain is controlled, the patient may be well enough to get up, or even to go home for a few weeks. Many will spend part of the morning in the dayroom where they may watch television, develop a new skill in occupational therapy, or chat with friends. Several hospices have a sitting room in which patients who are mobile enough can entertain their friends and take tea provided by voluntary workers.

So often I have heard it said, 'Terminal care? I couldn't do that, it must be awfully depressing.' That this popular picture of a hospice as a gloomy house full of agonized corpse-like people is not accurate is a tribute to the quality of the nursing. Although extreme illness is treated with horror and people avoid even looking at it, [189] it is often a positive force, binding people together and bringing out the best in them. It is not a question of getting hardened to suffering – one always remains vulnerable. If one person is to receive comfort, someone else has to give it up. Merely staying beside someone who is struggling with physical deterioration and mental anguish can be very painful. But this pain can be a rewarding experience, because of the comfort such fellowship brings to the patient.

Although some patients are in the hospice for only a few days, others may spend much longer in the ward. To benefit fully from the care a hospice gives, some patients need to be there for several weeks. Inevitably the staff will make friends with them, so that a series of bereavements for the staff cannot be avoided. If a much loved patient dies, there is a cloud over the whole ward for a while. To support the staff and to develop their own insight, group meetings are held to discuss these matters. For one person alone it might well prove too much, but with the strength of a whole caring community, it is easy. This is the main reason why specialist hospices are needed: the individual's confidence can be sustained by the group which will also guide his attitude to his work.

To watch someone coming to terms, in his own special way, with an unbearable situation, is a very great privilege. Here more than anywhere else a good nurse can give valuable help. On their death beds many men mature wonderfully. Priorities fall into place, tolerance and courage may grow in the most unlikely soil and more amazing still is the serenity which so often comes to one from the dying.

Much of the work of those caring for the dying is to prevent anything arising which may hinder this growth in the patient's being. He must be free from pain, but still alert; he must be told as much of the truth about his condition as he can cope with, but no more; he must be encouraged to turn his attention away from himself, and must be given a clean example of real service.[137]

When a man's responsibilities drop away, either by reason of physical weakness or of senile dementia, there remains a great beauty which has been covered by busyness – or laziness – for many a year. Death removes the covers: this unmasking can be a thrilling revelation.

When people say that they would find the care of the dying depressing, I wonder whether they are not denying expression to that very part of their nature which could give the most to others. Nurses or doctors who get elated or depressed with their patients are not considering what the patients may need from them. It follows that such feelings must be self-centred. This kind of 'involvement' may well render a person useless. Just so she who grieves with him, suffers with him, 'feels for him' or does anything but serve him.

To see a man's needs and to minister to them efficiently and considerately requires a measure of detachment. This is not – as is commonly supposed – a cold thing. Far from it! – it is an indispensable pre-requisite of love. Surges of emotion take your attention off the person in need on to yourself. However, if some situation is very moving another trap is to try to conceal your feelings. When you consider it, such suppression is untruthful. It is better to keep a level head if you can, but if you cannot, at least do not be dishonest about it!

I remember one family who were overwhelmed with gratitude because the nurse who imparted bad news to them also cried with them. 'How wonderful,' they said afterwards, 'that she cared so much.' The significant thing, however, was that she *stayed* with them in spite of her own sorrow and embarrassment.

This love is essential in caring for the dying. In a general ward, there is usually so much one can do for the patients that the duty to be with them and the pure giving entailed in listening to them can be dismissed as an encumbrance. But to provide the dying with masses of hospital equipment and drugs, and no love, is like offering a pot of gold to a starving man buried in sovereigns.

The right attitude to the dying, then, is neither that of a vivisector, nor that of an indulgent granny, but is one of esteem, of reverence, of loving kindness. This is a tall order, certainly, but it is a worthy aim. In this setting one hopes the patient may be able to approach death like the Chinese poet Po Chü-i, who wrote:

> Within my breast no sorrows can abide,
> I feel the great world's spirit through me thrill

And as a cloud I drift before the wind,
Or with the random swallow take my will.

As underneath the mulberry tree I dream,
The water-clock drips on, and dawn appears:
A new day shines o'er wrinkles and white hair,
The symbols of the fullness of my years.

If I depart, I cast no look behind;
If still alive, I still am free from care.
Since life and death in cycles come and go,
Of little moment are the days to spare.

Thus strong in faith I wait and long to be
One with the pulsings of Eternity.

Poem transcribed by L. Cranmer-Byng[128]

The Patient Dies

The vigil of relatives and friends, or just one of the hospice staff, must be discreetly supervised to prevent its being a traumatic experience. People feel helpless beside the dying because they do not realize that what counts is their presence, not their activity. They may feel guilty because the mind plays with irrelevant thoughts, taking attention off the dying person. They should be encouraged to touch the patient – hold his hand for instance – for this will be one of his last channels of reassurance. To the last he can be assumed to hear all that is said. Often a flicker of a smile or a faint squeeze of a finger will confirm that the message has been received. In searching for the appropriate message, people commonly turn to the traditional prayers and scriptures of the Church; the *Nunc Dimittis* for instance:

Lord, now lettest thou thy servant depart in peace, according to thy word: For mine eyes have seen thy salvation, which thou has prepared before the face of all people. – Luke 2: 29–31

Distress in the last hour is rare and the fear of it is a morbid twist in our culture. The idea of suffering may well be projected on to a person by distressed spectators who are in fact dreading their own imminent bereavement. There is, on the contrary, almost always a rather beautiful giving-in. The person withdraws serenely and willingly, as gently as an ocean liner slips away from the quayside. Sometimes there may be a brief period of complete lucidity.

In her booklet *Care of the Dying* (see Bibliography) Dr Cicely Saunders wrote:

Some have said to me that they hoped 'it would be in their sleep', and this is something we can promise with little fear that we will be wrong. We must be ready to use sedation for the occasional patient who feels that he is choking or suffocating but almost always unconsciousness precedes death.

3. Teamwork

Modern doctors and nurses cannot work in isolation. They need a host of other ancillary workers. Gradually the doctor's role is emerging as that of a team leader, the coordinator of what Sir Theodore Fox called 'The Greater Medical Profession',[120] a term embracing doctors in all specialties, with nurses, physiotherapists, occupational therapists, social workers, laboratory technicians, radiographers, speech therapists and so on.

Who Are The Team?

If robots could replace men, A would look after B, and their roles would be distinct. But in real life nothing is so clear-cut. We have the situation in which a dying man's needs must be met, and everyone who contributes to or benefits from this situation is one of the team. Everyone involved has the opportunity to care and to learn. Each can be of help to the other. The team seen in this way – as including everyone who is contributing to the situation – becomes a much more alive, intelligent and human concept. It will include not only the hospital staff and family doctor team, but also the relatives and friends of the patient and, note this, the patient himself. How this can work, I will illustrate with the story of a Mrs N.

This lady in her forties had come from the West Indies with four of her older children so that they could be well educated and gain professional qualifications. After a few

34

years she was found to have a breast cancer. The breast was removed, and so were the ovaries in an effort to arrest the malignant process. Unfortunately, however, in her case this failed, and so did radiotherapy. The cancer spread to her liver and bones, making her feel very ill, and giving rise to great pain. When she came into our care, she commented, 'I had an operation for my breast and now my liver is big,' clearly indicating that she appreciated her diagnosis. She said she would love to see her children in Grenada, but didn't suppose she ever would now, though her passport and vaccinations were up to date.

Having relieved her pain, we made tentative inquiries as to how the money for a flight home to Grenada might be found. One by one we met the family and heard of her hopes for each. She said the oldest boy had turned out to be a 'bad lot' and had little to do with his mother, leaving her very concerned that the other two boys should not fall into similar ways. In particular the younger, B., was beginning to keep bad company. So when we pointed out that she was too weak to fly alone, she chose young B. to be her companion on the plane, reasoning that if she could get him away from London he could work on his father's farm in moral safety. Most of the money was raised by her son named L., and her daughter – who were both now working. The last £100 was kindly contributed by the National Society for Cancer Relief.

The complications were phenomenal. There was the night Mrs N. panicked and thought she would die before seeing home again; the cajoling of the customs to let through her two litre-bottles of heroin mixture!; the forklift to get her wheelchair on board the plane, and finally the losing of young B. in the air terminal, which delayed the flight.

We received a triumphant letter from Grenada some weeks later. She had pain again but obviously considered it unimportant. A fortnight later she died, just three days

35

after seeing her second daughter married in Grenada. Then the following September her son L. turned up at the hospice asking for work as a ward orderly, because he said it seemed a good place to be. When he moved on six months later, he told me that it was the first job from which he had never taken a day off.

Now who, in this story, was caring for whom? The decisions were all Mrs N.'s, every stage being discussed frankly with her. This is what I mean by a team approach. Life presented a problem, and all the people involved contributed what they could to deal with it responsibly.

'In giving himself time to meet his patient thus, the doctor will so often find that he himself gains more than he gives. It is from the dying that we learn to care for the dying.'[328] All that distinguishes the patient from the rest of the team is that his role in the play is that of dying.

In Britain today the patient is frequently told nothing about his diagnosis – he may even be told lies – yet his closest relatives are nearly always told. This is a hopelessly mechanical way of doing things, since the first person to be told should obviously be the one most able to take it. The patient may be the strongest member of the family, and may need to help them to accept the situation. Far from being supported by strong family relationships, however, the dying man often finds himself cut off by a wall of deception. The family are one moment preparing and planning for a world without him in it, and the next are talking about 'when you get better'. This can be very hard on a husband or wife who for decades has shared all troubles with the patient.[19] If this situation has been allowed to arise, it may be necessary to break down these barriers, very gently, to enable the couple to say their farewells. It is important to say goodbye. A conspiracy of silence will worsen the dying person's sense of isolation and stores up later emotional problems for the bereaved.[132] On the other hand of course, many patients will make it clear that they don't want to think about disease at all, and will leave everything to the doctor. This is just as valid, but at least the patient should be given the opportunity to choose which approach he would like to take.

Some relatives will be very obviously part of the caring side of the team, some will equally obviously be patients along with the dying man, and yet others will alternate between the two roles. It may be that they will need to be put up in the hospital overnight – as when they are too distressed to return home alone, or when they want to be close at hand if death is imminent.

While it would not be appropriate for them to read the patient's notes, which are worded for trained eyes only, relatives should be kept clearly in the picture – usually by a ward sister. If given the chance, they will have so many questions: Did he ask if he had cancer yesterday? What was he told? Why was his blood transfusion stopped? Do our visits tire him? How long has he to live now? To the extent that they are also patients, relatives need to be cared for as well. For this reason one or two hospices have a 'relatives' day off' when visiting of all but the most severely ill patients is discouraged. This releases the visitor who feels it is his duty to be with his loved one as much as possible, so that he never gets out. Visiting is otherwise unrestricted, of course, and this gives rise to no problems for the nursing staff.[175]

In the next three chapters I shall consider the contributions of all the other members of the team who constitute the 'Greater Medical Profession', and if one is fortunate enough to be supported by the goodwill of an army of voluntary workers, they also have a most valuable part to play. It may be economical to have a full-time organizer to recruit and deploy this help. I remember Mrs B., an old lady with extensive bone cancer whose hair had fallen out as a side-effect of some of the treatment she had been given. She spent Christmas Day covered in blushes and giggles because a hairdresser produced a wig for her, splendidly permed. It is worthwhile to keep a stock of wigs, spectacles, magnifying glasses, hearing aids and such like – discarded by ex-patients – for the purpose of helping present ones to live their last few weeks of life more fully. It would take too long to get new ones from the social services.

When unpleasant symptoms are under control and the patient is able to return home from hospital for a while, then a social worker can be the liaison between the two and can help to deal with the economic consequences of a disease which has wiped out a person's earning capacity.[28] All civil and financial worries should be resolved before he dies.

But there are bigger problems than this. One question always asked when someone is admitted to a hospital is 'What's your religion?' Many of the 'nominal C. of E.' group lapsed after the war, while several have said to me, 'I believe in Jesus, but I wouldn't go to church.' Nearly all of them appreciate a visit from a clergyman. Provided he is a familiar figure in the wards, his approach will not be accorded any dark significance. Ideally there should be a full-time hospital chaplain, whose role is that of another listener, who is particularly in tune with crises of conscience. The actual sectarian bent of the minister/priest/rabbi involved in such work is largely irrelevant provided he is obviously a clergyman and can listen. Once a particular cleric is found to be helpful, he is a very important member of the team caring for the dying. He should be consulted whenever possible, and such medical information as he needs confided in him,[423] for the patient may choose to speak frankly to any member of the team – ward sister, doctor, chaplain, social worker or physiotherapist.[88] And if he were to ask about his diagnosis or prognosis, uninformed embarrassed confusion may silence for ever the question which carries the most potential for relief of the patient's uncertainty, frustration and fears.

In other words, the doctor's ivory tower is crumbling. And so it should if the physical and spiritual comfort of the patient is in question. Medicine, after all, is no longer in charge of the situation: death is taking over. No amount of professional tradition, etiquette or administrative difficulty, however heavy, can be an excuse for failing to minister to the self-evident needs of a dying man.

A man who wishes to prepare himself for death may need help. Which member of the team he chooses to confide in is entirely his own affair. More senior staff need not be offended because he did not speak to them. Indeed, if none of the hospital staff wins his trust, they should be ready to call in the family doctor or district nurse, who may have known the patient for many years. At the end of one of his excellent papers Professor John Hinton stressed this need for good communication between all the people concerned with the care of a person who is dying.[158]

When the patient goes home cured, his thankfulness overlooks gaps in the service, but when he is dying the result will be a shambles if the team is not pulling together. The situation puts a stress on the system. If it is a traditional system, with a godly and unapproachable consultant whose potential team is divided by professional jealousies and jargon, who never meet together and communicate infrequently, then this stress will reveal the deficiencies. Someone will suffer.

Mr F. was dying at home in the care of the Macmillan Service. He was an old war horse who had been a very fine leather craftsman in his prime. Both he and his wife were rather deaf, so they barked at one another. He delivered stentorian orders to her and to anyone else in the house, with an iron will that never faltered. One day I took him home from the clinic because the ambulances had let us down. We had to heave him out of the car and help him across a square, surrounded by council rent-slabs, to reach the tower block in which he lived. His pyjama trousers began to slip.

'Tie me pants up!' he ordered.

'What?' his wife asked.

'Me pants! Me pants! Get them fastened.'

'Oh damn you.' And she knelt before him to retie the

cord, but it was not to his liking. He aimed a clout at her but she deftly evaded it, evidently being well-practised. We proceeded a few more paces and his trousers fell down completely. Fascinated faces appeared in windows all round the square as he stood, bottom half naked, shaking with rage and bellowing abuse at the poor woman until she hitched his trousers up again.

He wanted desperately to stay in control of the situation around him, and to stay proudly independent. In spite of a troublesome colostomy he had firmly left the hospital which had been treating his rectal carcinoma, and refused to return to their out-patients. 'I wouldn't be in this mess but for them,' he said. After all, it was inconceivable that *he* could be going to pieces, such disasters could only be imposed from outside.

When we first met him he certainly was in a mess. Incontinent of urine, with a leaky colostomy and bedsores, he was a pathetic figure. His wife, obedient but resentful and short of breath, also worried us. Our district nursing sister visited them and reorganized the colostomy bags with a better adhesive. She catheterized* him and taught his wife how to manage the bedsores.

Socially acceptable again, he found a new lease on life, and demanded rehabilitation. This proved too much for his district nurse, and in a case conference his GP grieved that domiciliary physiotherapy was not available. Eventually this need was filled by enthusiastic youngsters from the local parish who were sent by the vicar to help Mr F. to walk.

The social worker made the acquaintance of Mrs F. in the clinic, with a view to helping her in bereavement. In spite of their explosive relationship it transpired that these two were deeply devoted in their own odd way. When she was told he had only a few weeks of life left she became very quiet and soft. I never saw her yell at him again: his every imperious whim was carried out at once.

As he became weaker, however, the nursing became

*See p. 82.

heavier and heavier for his wife. I watched her jugular pulse and ankle oedema with increasing concern. But when I put it to him that his wife's heart was failing he just reassured me that there was no such problem. 'She's coping marvellous,' he announced. Then one morning I found her gasping for breath and decided that he really must come into the hospice to give her a rest. Mr F. was adamant, however: he was going to die at home.

'Before or after your wife?' I ranted. That was Saturday. Later in the day the GP tried, with no more success than I had had. On Sunday the vicar went in and spoke of the duty to give in and trust. But on Monday the last straw was added by Sister, who turned on the blarney as only an Irish nun can. Making a number of conditions and provisos he agreed to come in, and in fact died contentedly in the hospice a few days later. His wife's health was saved in the nick of time, and she kept up her friendship with us by becoming a voluntary worker, making tea for the out-patient clinic. Bereavement follow-up was thus easy.

Only with the closest teamwork was this outcome possible.

The Roles Overlap

Clearly the roles of doctor, priest and nurse are not going to be in neat compartments, for at times they will be completely interchangeable.[243] To be instantly responsive to the patient's needs one requires nurses who can alter the dosage of drugs, recognize when to give a wide range of 'when necessary' prescriptions, and insert a urinary catheter. One needs doctors who can also be spiritual advisers, and clergymen who can competently impart a grave prognosis. It is the widening of the scope of one's work, closer to the traditional role of the old-time family doctor, which is the principal attraction in care of the dying.

It is a sphere in which one will inevitably find nurses teaching doctors, and vice versa. The needs of the situa-

41

tion are so obvious that petty divisions become unimportant. An example of good communication in one hospice is the 'pink sheet' to be found in each patient's notes. On this are recorded any significant comments made by a patient which may reveal the progress of his growing insight into his condition. Any member of the staff may write on this sheet or use it for reference – nurses, social workers, physiotherapists, chaplains or doctors.

Nurses in general hospitals may be uneasy about some of the doctor's decisions in the care of dying patients: Why were Mrs Whatsit's antibiotics stopped? Why can't Mr Overthere be left in peace instead of having all those tubes pushed in every orifice? Nurses need help with what to say to the dying patient[251] and what is to be their own attitude to death. The best person to deal with these problems is often a chaplain who is versed in medical ethics. Diffident nurses who will not question the medical staff can go to him, and he can help the two groups to communicate with each other over the nurses' ethical dilemmas.

A Partnership of Equals

The following is part of an essay dictated by Enid Henke,[156] a lady dying of motor neurone disease who was herself too weak to write:

A friend and I were considering life and its purpose. I said, even with increasing paralysis and loss of speech I believed there was a purpose for my life but I was not sure what it was at that particular time ... After a while my friend said, 'It must be hard to be the wounded Jew when by nature you would rather be the Good Samaritan.'

It is hard: It would be unbearable were it not for my belief that the wounded man and the Samaritan are inseparable. It was the helplessness of the one that brought out the best in the other and linked them together.

In reflecting on the parable I am particularly interested in the fact that we are not told the wounded man recovered. I have always assumed that he did but it now occurs to me that even if he did not recover the story would still stand as a perfect example of true neighbourliness. You will remember that the story concludes with the Samaritan* asking the inn-keeper to take care of the man, but he assures him of his own continuing interest and support: so the innkeeper becomes linked ...

Enid was another patient who, one felt, was caring for the staff while they cared for her. In exploring the answer to my question 'Who is caring for whom?' I remembered how often patients may care for one another, with re-assurance, example and friendship. Then I remembered how patients like Enid can care for the staff by being considerate of their feelings, and by just accepting ser-vice.[356] And finally there came to mind all the ways the staff can help one another by discussion and the sharing of experience and troubles.[68]

This, then, is the team which stands ready to serve and to encourage the dying patient. Though they work in much the same way as with recuperating patients, the emphasis is different. Always before them, the focal point and perfectly appropriate conclusion to their whole work, is a special moment – perhaps months away, perhaps to-morrow – when the patient will die. To this moment all their efforts will be directed, that it may be peaceful, joy-ful and contented.

*Luke 10:29–37.

4. The Pains of Death

'In birth there is pain, decay brings pain, disease is painful, death is painful.' So mused the Buddha in his famous sermon on the End of Suffering. But is all this pain really necessary?

Pain in the Body

Once again I will stress that for dying patients we should be treating symptoms, not diseases. Pain is the symptom we usually fear the most, particularly if we hear the much dreaded diagnosis of 'cancer'. Indeed, without careful treatment 40% of patients with cancer might have severe pain.[373] Good treatment should anticipate pain, because if pain returns before the next dose of analgesics, it will be all the harder to control.[50] If they are given regularly, the dose of analgesics can be kept low (see Table 1, p. 49), though there should be no hesitation in giving sufficiently large doses.

I remember one old Glaswegian patient who found his own optimum dose. He came to us from one of H.M. Prisons, with the pain-killers for his lung cancer in a sealed bag. He was a guest of H.M. for being drunk and disorderly, but the prison doctors had found that he had only a short time to live. In the ambulance he opened the medicines, and finding that one was liberally laced with gin he swigged from it with delight. On arrival he rather unsteadily handed me the empty bottle, and I realized with horror that he had consumed about fifteen times the

44

normal dose of morphine. I watched to see if he would lapse into a coma, but all that arose was a happy smile and 'Och, it sure got rid o' the pain, doc.'

What must be avoided is the giving of analgesics 'when necessary' (or 'PRN' as doctors say, from the Latin *pro re nata*). This means that the pain gradually builds up until the patient asks a nurse for relief. She will tell the ward sister, who will have to break off from her other work to give an injection. The drug brings drowsiness with pain relief and the patient remains dully half-aware until he cries out again for morphine. Then someone says, 'I suspect he's getting addicted.' For a dying patient, however, there is no maximum dose of an analgesic drug.

A Mr H. told me he had been 'in agony for three months'. I thought he was romancing until I examined him with attention, and found how intensely tender were the cancer deposits in his ribs. Even breathing hurt him and any movement produced whimpers of misery from great pain. He had been receiving powerful opiate analgesics throughout the three months, but the dose had been kept down for fear of addiction. Two days after coming to the hospice he was sitting up, relaxed and smiling. Pain of the kind that Mr H. had endured can seem to fill the whole universe, leaving the patient conscious of little else.

If pain is properly controlled, the patient will never feel it again. He will ask if the medicines are really necessary any more, because the pain has gone.[325] Then it may be possible for him to return home and have his pain control organized as an out-patient.[315] In the clinic, medical and social support can be combined at the time when it is most needed and the patient can die comfortably at home.

Of course there are many valuable ways of controlling pain which do not involve morphine. Aspirin, PR spray and rubbing with oil of wintergreen or rubifacients like Balmosa or Algipan are all helpful, not to mention alcohol, which is a first class sedative and an excellent adjuvant in the relief of pain. But if pain is severe then we have to turn to the opiate family of drugs – morphine, heroin, phenazocine (Narphen), dipipanone (Diconal), oxycodone and the codeines. Few of the hospices still use heroin, which is now illegal in most countries, because it has actions identical to those of morphine (at least as far as pain-killing is concerned).[381] Its only advantage is that it is more soluble, which helps if injections are having to be used. British experience therefore suggests that there is no justification for recent moves to get heroin re-introduced into the USA.[131] The difference for the patients comes not so much from the magic chemical used as from the intelligence with which it is used.[220] Morphine doses have to be one and a half times the heroin dose to be equally potent.

Doctors who otherwise pride themselves on careful diagnosis followed by rational and precise treatment so often seem to sink into a mire of mythology and emotions when faced with a dying patient. Science goes to the wind and superstition takes over.

Patients are ignored when they most need attention, deceived when they most need someone with the courage to face their predicament with them and, worst of all, left in pain because the doctor fears to use the analgesics readily available to him.[169]

Morphine is believed to be dangerous and addictive, to shorten patients' lives, to be hallucinogenic, to be cumulative in some mysterious way and to be needed in larger and larger doses because patients 'develop tolerance to it'. It is believed to be euphoriant (some hospitals even call their variation on the Brompton Cocktail 'Mist E' for euphoria) and to have a long duration of action – six, eight or even twelve hours.

Let us look at these beliefs individually. All are wrong!

Compared with many other drugs in everyday use – e.g. digoxin, insulin – the opiates are remarkably safe.[380] The name 'dangerous drugs' does not apply to their role in the field of medicine, but to their rather different use in Piccadilly Circus. The lethal dose of morphine is not known for certain but is probably around half a gram. There are exceptions, of course: a patient with an unstable blood pressure just after a heart attack, or a patient with emphysema who has been breathless with blue lips for a long time, should not be given large doses of opiates. But for the majority of patients dying with a painful cancer, impairment of breathing is a negligible side-effect of the opiates, sometimes useful in the treatment of breathlessness, but never hastening their demise.

Far from it. A patient distressed by pain and terrified of dying becomes rapidly exhausted and dies quickly and badly. With the proper use of opiate analgesia he will be peaceful and comfortable, living longer and dying with dignity.

How often do I hear otherwise highly observant doctors saying, 'I'm holding back the opiates to the very end, so that they will still be effective.' They fail to see the agonized patient to whom they are giving only paracetamol and they fail to observe the effects of morphine when it is given. We have had patients on four-hourly morphine or heroin for periods of over two years. They did not need steadily increasing dosage. Attempts to reduce the dose by 5 or 10 mg resulted in a return of the pain: the morphine was *titrated* against the pain to a point which exactly held it. Thereafter no change was needed unless the pain changed. If for some reason the pain goes away (e.g. after palliative radiotherapy or artificial strengthening of an unstable bone)[114] then the morphine can be tailed off and stopped. I have never known this process to present difficulties. Addiction is a myth. Certainly after weeks of administration of an opiate, a degree of physical dependence arises, so that sudden withdrawal results in sweating, goose pimples and panic, but this has nothing to do with addiction.[401] We do not say that patients get addicted to steroid drugs, but we know that they cannot be suddenly withdrawn. Addiction is a psychic phenomenon resulting from craving for a repeat of the 'high' obtained by pushing the opiate into a vein. Given orally or by intramuscular injection, opiates (heroin included) have no such effect. They are not even as euphoriant as two black coffees or a glass of champagne, and undue increase of dosage is experienced by the patient as drowsiness rather than psychedelia. If there is no 'high' there can be no addiction. The whole idea is a gremlin.

What the patients certainly may be craving for is an end to the pain. Few things could be more shocking than to hear a nurse say, 'Miss X keeps begging for her morphine. I think she's getting addicted, so we'll ask doctor to cut down the dose.' Look at the treatment card, and there it is: 'Morphine 10 mg IM, PRN.' Why IM (by injection) when it can be given by mouth? Injections hurt. But above all, why oh why 'PRN'? To treat continuous pain 'when necessary' means that in the doctor's opinion the patient should always earn his analgesia by having a little touch of agony first.[172] From the patient's point of view it means he is never free from pain for long. He tenses up against its return, so needs more morphine next time. He lives in fear of pain and can never forget that he has, for example, cancer. Fear and anxiety lower his pain threshold dramatically, so he needs even more morphine next time. The big dose makes him drowsy, he thinks he is dying, and he is terrified. Now no amount of morphine will ever control the pain. This is how the myth of 'tolerance' arose.[376] (I hear that in Piccadilly the addicts need more and more drugs to have the same psychic effect. That is totally irrelevant to the use of opiates as analgesics.)

Of 339 patients who died of cancer in our care, only one third ever needed injections. That means that two thirds were able to take an analgesic mixture within four hours of their death. Only two needed 150 mg oral morphine or its equivalent. 62% of those with pain never needed more than 60 mg morphine four-hourly by mouth: 35% never needed more than 20 mg[377] (Table 1).

But if pain is severe, it should not be tickled with half-hearted analgesia.[231] 100 mg morphine four-hourly by mouth is not an enormous dose – it is just the upper end of the usual normal range for cancer pain (the dose will be halved if injections are unavoidable). Failure to use

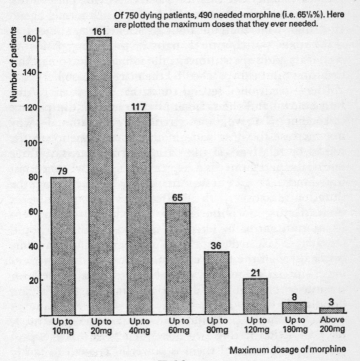

Of 750 dying patients, 490 needed morphine (i.e. 65⅓%). Here are plotted the maximum doses that they ever needed.

Table 1

adequate doses accounts for an awful lot of distressful dying.

Hallucinations are unusual. Just over 1% of our patients suffer this side-effect; and if they have it with one opiate, they do with any other, and with the group of drugs called opiate-antagonists. One may then be obliged to use methadone or other drugs with dissimilar molecules. What does cause hallucinations, nightmares, confusion, and even mania is the cocaine which tradition dictates be added to so many analgesic mixtures. It is a potent drug with many side-effects. It has not been shown to confer any substantial benefit.[275] Why then is it prescribed so widely? Because doctors lose their cool before a dying patient and fall back upon the myths and witchcraft of a former age.[375] It is high time that the light of science was allowed to shine upon the control of pain in the dying patient.[154] The fears and superstitions in the minds of doctors in this situation can be dispatched by the mace of reason.

I have mentioned several times that we give morphine four-hourly (and the same applies to heroin, dipipanone or codeine). To give it more frequently is irrational – why not increase the dose and give less inconvenience to the nurses or relatives? If the pain returns after, say, three hours, the patient needs a bigger dose which will then last four hours. To give it less frequently is cruel, since the duration of action of these drugs does not stretch to six hours. Giving morphine six-hourly condemns the patient to intermittent pain. This is so unnecessary that it should nowadays be classed as negligence. Should pain at any time break through the drug control, it must be dealt with at once – prescriptions of extra analgesics must be left for the nurses to use at their discretion. Some drugs which are popular have an even shorter duration. Pethidine,[231] dextromoramide (Palfium) and pentazocine (Fortral)[166] have an action lasting two hours or less in this group of patients, and none of them is powerful enough to tackle severe cancer pain. It is also our clinical impression that they have a higher incidence of side-effects than do other opiates. Another potent painkiller is methadone. This is not suitable for long-term use because it is cumulative,[165] unlike any of the opiate drugs, probably collecting in the brain.[272] It can be used when a patient with severe pain is lapsing into coma a day or two before death.[443] Then it will not have time to cumulate and its long duration of action means it need only be given eight-hourly. If the pain is less severe, then buprenorphine (Temgesic) 0.6 mg can be given 8–12 hourly – a convenient drug for use in a patient's home.[92]

If addiction, tolerance and hallucinations belong with the mythology of opiate treatment, there are two vital side-effects which do occur and are all too often ignored. The first is nausea which is frequent. Anti-emetics (drugs to control nausea) should always be given when opiates are administered on a regular basis. But the choice of anti-emetic is crucial. Chlorpromazine (Largactil) is too soporific for most patients and should be reserved for those who are so anxious that sedation is actually what is wanted. Prochlorperazine (Stemetil) and perphenazine (Fentazin) in small dosage – such as 5 mg four-hourly – are usually preferable.

The second side-effect of long-term opiate treatment *always* occurs, should be prevented and, not being so, causes more misery and additional ill-health to dying patients than almost any other factor. This is constipation.

All these pain-killing drugs are constipating and patients still form faeces even when they are not eating. Faeces are not formed only of left-over food but also of sloughed-off bowel wall. In Belsen they still had bowel-movements – that was the main way in which they lost weight. Yet how often do I hear 'He's not eating so he won't have his bowels opened will he?' In fact the patient may not be eating *because* he has had no bowel action for a week. Time and again we are asked to see patients in the Macmillan Service who have constipation bad enough to cause anorexia, vomiting or confusion.[224] One in ten of the patients referred to us for terminal care has constipation of such long standing that a complete faecal impaction has occurred, the bowel being jammed up with rock-solid material which has to be removed by hand.

A person who is emaciated with widespread cancer must still empty his bowels regularly. In the Macmillan Service we assume that anyone who is having an opiate analgesic (including codeine and DF 118) *will* be constipated. There is no point in waiting to see. So whenever we prescribe one of these drugs we routinely also give an aperient. For this kind of constipation the best drug, we have found, is Dorbanex Forte, 10 ml once or twice a day. Of course prevention is better than cure, but we also have a rule that on the third day with no bowel action nurses should give Dulcolax suppositories and if they don't work it should be an enema the next day. The relief this can bring to the patient is enormous.

When I say an enema, I do mean a real enema – not just a little Fletcher's rectal washout. They make me wonder if the nurse is afraid of getting her hands dirty. Someone who is really constipated – say only two or three bowel actions in the last month – will present obvious signs. The abdomen will be rather gassy and distended. The descending colon will be easy to feel. Bowel sounds will be continuous and often audible without a stethoscope. Rocks may be felt in the rectum.

There may be a continuous slight overflow of liquid faeces leaking past the obstruction. The anal muscles are stretched by the hard lumps and cannot close, so the patient complains of 'diarrhoea' because he may be incontinent of this overflow. So the doctor prescribes Lomotil and the situation gets worse. In such a situation there may be faeces palpable in the transverse colon or even in the caecum. That means 3ft 6in. of bowel all blocked.

So the patient cannot be said to have had his constipation relieved until the nurse has seen that length of faeces in the pan. Moving things up six inches by a rectal washout is clearly useless. A two-foot-long rubber tube is needed and a good pint of hot fluid, or the contents of at least two Fletcher's enemas, in order to stimulate the bowel from around the splenic flexure.

Dark tales are told of the occasional patient who died after a proper enema. Pay no heed. Far more die of constipation than ever did of enemas. Indeed, we recently had four patients referred to us in one month who were actually dying until given an enema.

If the analgesic dose needed to control a patient's pain

is rising unduly his situation needs overall assessment, remembering always that what matters is how the patient sees it, not what an outside observer makes of it. If the patient says it is agonizing, that is the assessment that really counts because no one else can share his way of experiencing it.[87] Pain is not simply a matter of electrical impulses travelling up particular nerves. It is an expression of the way the whole individual meets the events of his life.[108] Physical and mental suffering are closely interwoven and a division into bodily and mental pain is an artificial one.

Often the need for increasing quantities of analgesics is a sign that more sedatives or tranquillizers are required to raise the patient's threshold to the physical pain.

Long-standing relentless pain is almost a disease in itself, because of the devastating effects it has on the person. He cannot get away from it, it commands his attention, and yet it seems completely meaningless. Dr Lawrence LeShan likened the situation to a nightmare:

The person in pain is in the same formal situation; terrible things are being done to him and he does not know if worse will happen; he has no control and is helpless to take effective action; no time limit is given ... the patient lives during the waking state in the cosmos of the nightmare.[214]

Whether a person can be helped to *find* a meaning to his pain will be considered later, but certainly the judicious use of tranquillizers, combined with seeing doctors and nurses tackle his pain with confidence, can alleviate a great deal of distress and halt the rising need for pain-killers.

A variety of minor physical discomforts can, in combination, make it very much more difficult for the patient to override pain.

Everything which causes physical discomfort has to be dealt with: sore mouths and painful infections like boils and cystitis, for instance. Insomnia is also distressing. Sleeping tablets may be a help but it is necessary to inquire into the cause of the sleeplessness. Perhaps it is due to pain, which is often worse at night. In this case the analgesics have to be given regularly right round the clock, with a slightly higher dose at night.[150] A cough can also make sleep impossible, so a linctus should be available at the bedside. One of the worst enemies of sleep is anxiety. Alcohol or sedatives may have a place here, but nothing compares with a sympathetic listener. Then there are the obvious causes of insomnia that can easily be overlooked. If the patient is at home the person with whom he sleeps may be restless. If he is in hospital other patients may be noisy or the bed may be hard. (And see p. 79.)

Particular kinds of pain may require more specialized techniques instead of, or as well as, opiates. The surgical pinning of an unstable bone, for example, may give such dramatic relief that the procedure is worthwhile even in a patient who cannot survive for long. Although radiotherapy is no longer appropriate as a curative measure, an experienced radiotherapist can use his skill to bring about a reduction in the size of metastases which were causing pain or discomfort by the sheer pressure of their size. Techniques of nerve blocking are also being developed with moderate success, a skilled anaesthetist giving injections at various points along pain pathways to relieve acute and localized pain.[64]

Patients with brain tumours may suffer with severe headaches and nausea due to pressure from fluid collecting around the tumour. This kind of pain can be managed by a combination of approaches from 'physics, chemistry and biology'. Physics suggests that the fluid pressure can be lowered by raising the head of the bed 8–10 inches and providing a 'donkey' (see p. 80) at the patient's feet to prevent him sliding down the bed. A diuretic drug can be given which makes the patient pass more urine and thus lowers the fluid pressure in all his cells by chemical means. The activity of the cells themselves can be biologically modified by large doses of powerful steroid drugs (up to 4 mg dexamethasone, thrice daily). But if this condition typifies the need for a multiple approach to relief, it also illustrates the absolute necessity of knowing when to stop interfering. Steroids may make a dramatic difference for a while, the patient's unpleasant symptoms virtually disappearing. But it is the symptom of fluid pressure which is being relieved, not the tumour itself. This will continue to grow and, if the steroids are continued, pressure from the cancer will reproduce those symptoms (usually within a few weeks) and thus leave the patient as badly off as he was before, but carrying the additional burden of side-effects from steroid drugs which are no longer doing him any good.

Widespread aches and pains and loss of appetite are common among dying patients. They too can be dramatically helped by steroid drugs given in much smaller doses. 5 mg of prednisolone three times each day is not a large dose.[95] It can safely be given over quite a long period and can much increase the patient's sense of well-being.

Pain in the Mind

Specific physical symptoms produce, or may be the result of, characteristic attitudes of mind. A knowledge of what goes with what can often help us to help patients on two levels at once. Anxiety, for example, often goes with breathlessness, so relieving either will help with the other while coping with both will banish the whole syndrome. Depression often comes with nausea, weakness or loss of appetite, and once again an attack on all fronts simultaneously will often prove effective. If these afflictions are not relieved, the strain of keeping a stiff upper lip will usually prove too great, and when it does, the patient can feel humiliated. Disease itself cannot be humiliating because humiliation is a particular relationship between people and cannot therefore be caused by any *thing*. But illness can lead to relationships which feel humiliating to the patient and therefore good nursing must manifest respect for him and preserve his dignity whatever happens.

Pains in the mind are as various as the people they assail, but fear is something we are all vulnerable to, particularly when we are dying. If we are sensitive in our communication with dying patients, we can detect many of their fears and, more importantly, dispel many of the most grim. 'Why didn't you come earlier?' we say to the patient who approaches us for the first time when his disease has progressed far beyond the curable stage. Fear of mutilating operations and uncomfortable and frightening investigations and treatments is often the answer.

A patient's disease may itself give rise to bizarre but terrifying ideas. One man with cancer of the stomach developed a sore throat. Fortunately I discovered that he was afraid that the cancer was spreading up from below to strangle him and was able to reassure him that while the cancer was a fact that could not be avoided, the sore throat was a different and completely trivial matter. There are patients who dare not go to sleep in case they die, or who are afraid that if they sleep they may be thought dead and be buried alive. Reassurance can dispel this terrified insomnia. Other patients fear that their cancer will send them mad; that it is hereditary, infectious or simply dirty and disgusting.

Uncertainty about a diagnosis or prognosis often gives rise to more intolerable fear than does the grimmest certainty. A Mrs G. told us that she had been far more afraid when she suspected that she was dying than she was now that she had knowledge of the fact. A Miss P. had a bowel cancer which had been by-passed by a colostomy so that her bowels discharged themselves into a bag attached to an opening made through her abdomen. She had faced this major operation and traumatic adaptation and had lost two stones in weight yet, as I examined her abdomen, she said, 'There doesn't seem to be much wrong, does there, Doctor?' There was such questioning in this cautious probe that I sat down to listen. 'I don't understand about this colostomy,' she went on. 'Is it going to heal up?' No patient should be left with this kind of uncertainty.

Left unsure of what is happening or is likely to happen to them, patients are prey to all manner of terrors, particularly to the fear that when death itself comes it will be violent, with overwhelming pain or suffocation. In fact we find that pain nearly always subsides just before the end; the patient feels only an overwhelming drowsiness and dies in his sleep. These fears are ghosts which can be exorcized by anyone who will discuss them or refer them to the doctor. Whatever form they take, they are additional burdens on the dying patient and it is as much our duty to remove this burden as it is to remove his bodily pain.

Another mental pain to be considered is guilt. On a superficial level this can be felt by a patient who is incontinent or has a discharging ulcer which has a bad smell. The bed linen should be frequently changed, and the patient frequently reassured that those nursing him don't mind doing this. Infected ulcers can be treated remarkably effectively by injections of a mixture of penicillin and streptomycin,* provided that the patient is not so thin that the injections are too painful. The ulcers themselves can be rinsed or syringed clean with the solutions recommended for deep bedsores on p. 81, and the use of yoghurt as a dressing prevents further infection.

At a deeper level, a man may be burdened with feelings of guilt or incompleteness on looking back over a mediocre life. The disease may feel like a punishment. When one lady was told that she was dying she said, 'I get so depressed, you know: I've never done anyone any harm.'

Oddly enough, psychotherapists are very cautious about relieving people of this guilt, as we shall see in Chapter 10, for it has in it an element of truth.

Some patients are resentful of a disability which they feel is being imposed on them. They will blame the hospital, the drugs, or the doctors. For many people the idea of becoming dependent on others is unbearable. They

_____
*Crystamycin: one vial twice daily for about five days, until the smell subsides, then maintain on one dose per day.

need very matter-of-fact help, the worst of all things for them being pity, which implies a lower status. Under this kind of stress, some people regress to childish behaviour. One can make allowances for this if is understood as a defence-reaction to a situation they cannot bear to face. While he is strong enough, a person with this kind of personality will want all the physiotherapy and rehabilitation possible, particularly if he can make or do something useful for other people. Later, when dependence on others is thrust on him, every effort should be made to guard what remains of his autonomy. Nurses should remember not to chat to one another as if he were not there, doctors should not discuss his case over him, and everything done to him should be carefully explained beforehand.

A rather different kind of person will react to severe disease with intense grief. Suppose a hostile government were to announce that you had contravened a law that you had forgotten ever existed, and as a punishment stripped you of house and job and banished you. Family and friends would be lost forever behind an iron curtain. This is how some people feel when they are dying. The relatives who remain alive are only losing one person, but the dying man is losing everything: [6] his wife, his garden, the dog, his favourite chair and his own body.

'If only I could spend just a few days at home, in my little garden; it must be very beautiful now the spring is here.' So said Mrs R. who was completely bedridden. The pain from her cancer could only be controlled by an injection every four hours, supplemented by other analgesics given by mouth in between the injection times. She had thoroughly enjoyed her retirement, her home and her friends, and was very reluctant to lay them aside.

Another lady was miserable shortly after her last Christmas at home. I asked her what was depressing her. She cried a little and said, 'Nothing really, it's silly.' I said it was not silly, or she would not be crying. It transpired that she wanted just one more look at home. This was a tall order because she was too weak to get out of a chair, and was bleeding internally. However, I agreed to make plans for the projected trip and we fixed a day. Then I asked again what was depressing her. She clenched her fists and said, 'If I am ... ill ... again, can I come back here?' Her greatest pain was bereavement, but her greatest fear was loneliness.

This estrangement from the world haunts many people as they die, and they will try to compensate for it in various ways if they are not befriended. They may become over-demanding for fear of being left alone. They may complain vociferously about relatively minor pains as a respectable way of attracting attention. It is always worth while asking yourself, when somebody complains of pain, whether he is trying to communicate some other need to you as well. Careful listening to the complaint will reveal if this is so. Loneliness is particularly likely to produce this 'social pain' in a patient,[318] and so is worry about how the family will manage without him. Thus it can be seen that the social worker and the occupational therapist have a part to play in the relief of pain.

Social Pain

It is vital to maintain some kind of social life right to the end, for facing the unknown alone and friendless is a frightening prospect. One lady in a hospice said to me, 'You can talk to people more here. There everybody walked away from me.' When we do not walk away we share some of the pain. We may not understand, we cannot prevent the hard thing that is happening, but what really counts to the dying person is that someone cares enough to try. This was well expressed by Dr Ronald Welldon, shortly before his own death:

... as the realistic hopes of curative treatment diminish, the human or personal factors of relationship, motivation and emotion assume an importance which may not have been so obvious at a more optimistic stage. It becomes so much more tolerable to face intolerable aspects of a disease process, of oneself, and of life, if one can do so in the company of at least one other person, who is himself prepared to share something of this intolerability. Such a person does not necessarily have to hold a medical degree, but it helps. The person in the best position to help is still most frequently the family doctor, who has ready access to the patient as a member of a particular social group, with its various resources.[406]

There have been several occasions when, try as we might, we could not control a patient's pain while he was at home, but found it easy once he had been admitted to the hospice. No doubt the patient's improved condition would be partly due to his feeling safer, but we have also detected another factor. I remember the dramatic change in one gentleman whose wife was extremely anxious and fussed him a lot. 'Did he really have no pain at all after coming into the hospice?' I asked the ward sister. 'None,' she replied, 'well, except when his wife visited – then he always had it for a while.' One person's tension and anticipatory grief[318] can be communicated to another. Sometimes these situations can be improved by a social worker helping people to deepen their insight into their conduct, but sometimes the vicious circle can only be broken by rescuing a person into a totally different environment. 3·5% of admissions to the hospice from our Home Care Service are for this reason alone. One of the main reasons for our failure to control some people's pain was because there was a strong social element in it, but they still refused to be admitted to the hospice because of a feeling that they couldn't do without the problem relative.

It may not always be the relatives whose behaviour is causing distress. The patient's failure to accept his helplessness may be the problem. Again, it may be possible to help the patient to see what he is doing. As Dr Cicely Saunders once said:

Dependence on others is not the worst evil that can happen to us, and there are tremendous possibilities in accepting and sharing. Suffering is part of the whole of life, and although I spend my whole time trying to relieve it, I know what gains it brings to patient and family alike and what an immense deepening there so often is in their relationships.

The Greatest Pain of All

Mental and social pain are not so called fancifully. They can manifest as physical pain, complained of as such by the patient. It is when this fails to respond to ordinary medication that one is alerted to the deeper origin of the pain.

To be put in a position where one can be instrumental in relieving these various pains is a delight. The wonderful way so many people surmount their problems and fears makes one feel very humble. What is even more humbling is to realize that there is another pain, which we cannot treat, afflicting ourselves as well as our patients. In a few instances this 'spiritual pain', as we call it, can also present as an apparently physical complaint. It should certainly be considered if pain seems intractable.

Physical pains we suffer alone; mental and social pains, particularly grief, affect the whole circle of our acquaintances. But the greatest pain of all, a pain of the spirit, is as great as mankind. It is the pain of a prodigal son.*

Your pain is the breaking of the shell that encloses your understanding.
Even as the stone of the fruit must break, that its heart may stand in the sun, so must you know pain.
And could you keep your heart in wonder at the daily miracles of your life, your pain would not seem less wondrous than your joy;
And you would accept the seasons of your heart, even as you have always accepted the seasons that pass over your fields.
And you would watch with serenity through the winters of your grief.
Much of your pain is self-chosen.

*Luke 15:11–32.

It is the bitter potion by which the physician within you heals your sick self.

Therefore trust the physician, and drink his remedy in silence and tranquillity:

For his hand, though heavy and hard, is guided by the tender hand of the Unseen.

Kahlil Gibran: *The Prophet*

5. 1,000 Patients Dying at Home

Dying persons gain so much by being cared for by an affectionate family; they are better able to maintain themselves as individuals. Remaining at home, not swallowed up in the possible anonymity of the dying hospital patient, they need not doubt they are still part of the family. While among their family, they do not consider themselves as hulks awaiting the end, as long as they can participate, even in a limited role.
– Professor John Hinton's Pelican book, *Dying*, p.153

Every year over 40,000 people in Britain die at home, the majority suffering no great hardship.[413] For the minority, however, pressing needs do emerge. These were well documented by the Marie Curie Memorial Foundation and the Queen's Institute of District Nursing who carried out a joint survey in 1952 in order to know where to deploy the resources of the new Marie Curie Fund. Some 7,050 patients were involved in this painstaking and detailed research work, and most of its findings are still relevant today.[230] The needs for hospices and convalescent homes, for cancer education, for the coordinating of social work agencies, and for home helps were clearly seen. There was also an urgent need for night nurses.

The Foundation lost no time in implementing the findings. Their first hospice was opened in the same year – the Tidcombe Hall Home in Tiverton, Devon. The Area Welfare Grant Scheme made money available to district nurses for the urgent needs of cancer patients. They also began recruiting nurses who could act as 'sitters-in' to give relatives who were caring for patients with cancer adequate time for sleep and recreation. Introduced in 1958, the 'Day and Night Nursing Service' now employs the services of over 2,000 nurses. They are accessible through local Health Departments. In the words of the report – 'there are all kinds of attention which the patient requires (at night), including giving nourishment, adjusting the air-ring and pillows, helping him during the hours of restlessness and giving a sedative ...' To this one could add the giving of pain-killing injections if they are necessary.

Surveys of state services for the dying usually conclude that they are inadequate,[119] sometimes sadly so.[240] For example, when the family doctor is off duty he will often be replaced by a locum who probably knows nothing of the patient's history. When a patient is discharged from hospital it may be days or weeks before the family doctor is informed. In some areas it may be difficult to find the patient a hospital bed when urgently needed, and all over the country home helps and meals-on-wheels are usually in short supply. Even worse, the services which are available are not coordinated.[51] There may be no one connected with the family who is aware of the various available state and voluntary services, and they do not know whom to ask.

The Macmillan Service

The philosophy and organization of a domiciliary service for the dying in East London will be described, and then the practical aspects of patient care.

In 1973 a nurse and a doctor from St Joseph's Hospice in Hackney began to visit dying patients at home. The needs revealed were almost overwhelming. Great gaps in the provisions of the Health Services in a big city became immediately evident. Since that time several Health Districts have established night nursing services, but many still have not. The GP deputizing system is better than no doctor at all, but no substitute for someone who knows the patient's history and family. Lack of home support and poor symptom control lead families to panic and beg the doctor to hospitalize a dying person, and make hospital staff reluctant to discharge dying patients.[237] Yet in many hospital wards to die is an intimidating prospect,[73] for there is still a tendency to avoid the dying and to offer only sympathy for their symptoms. No one has time for these patients, largely because the staff feel helpless.

Two recent debates have suggested ways this situation could be tackled. The first is the growing interest shown in the French 'Hospital-at-Home' system.[59] Hospital-type of care, it has been found with many diseases, can be provided in a patient's home with telephone links to the base manned by specialist staff. That brings us to the second debate. Increasingly we are seeing the emergence of 'Clinical Nurse Specialists'[96] well able to manage certain types of care with only occasional back-up from a doctor.[7] Could not these two developments help the dying?[82]

To meet some of these needs the Macmillan Service was established at St Joseph's Hospice in 1975. The basic philosophy of this Service has been pragmatic: if you want it done properly, do it yourself. There is a tendency to see care of the dying as being mainly counselling and advising. It is not. Much of the Health Service is plagued by the profusion of advising chiefs and the paucity of working injuns. We also feel that to earn the right to a patient's confidence, one must first serve him in a concrete way. Trust must be deserved and won by giving families real support. Such support cannot be given 9 a.m. to 5 p.m., or stop short at a job demarcation.

Over the first three years of its working, 1,000 patients died in the care of the Macmillan Service. The lion's share went to patients with cancers of the lung (322), breast (153), bowel (97) and stomach (93). The average length of time for a patient to be under the Macmillan Service was about 60 days. Before they died 354 patients had to be admitted to the hospice, for a variety of reasons (Table 2). Of these, 31 actually spent less than a day in the hospice

	NUMBER OF PATIENTS OUT OF 1,000
Short stay for a rest	52
Caring relative exhausted or fell ill	120
Caring relative panicking	47
Caring relative in danger of losing job	8
Patient living alone: too weak to cope	76
Patient needing heavy sedation	28
Admitted for treatment, but deteriorated	22
Social component to the pain	13
Family rejecting the patient	13
Bowel obstruction	8
Diarrhoea	8
Patient asked to be admitted	8
Bleeding a problem	5
Paralysis	4
Family feud blew up	3

Table 2: Main Reasons for Admission to the Hospice

and a similar number were there for less than 48 hours before they died. It can be seen from the table that the reasons for admission are nearly always social, seldom medical. There is no good medical reason why people who are dying of cancer should not be at home, provided someone can look after them. Even if there is no one to care at home – and 121 of our patients lived alone, 32 of them with nobody but the Macmillan nurse calling in – proud independence can be maintained until the patient is bedbound. Even then, some refused to be admitted and died comfortably, if alone, in their own bed. One man's concept of death with dignity would not suit us all. There is a temptation to try to make people conform to stereotyped conduct. But one person will want to be sedated, another will regard being alert as his first priority; one will want to be pampered by nurses, another to fight his cancer to the last. It is often necessary to discuss this with the patient so that his aims can guide our therapy.

X-rays and blood tests are taken in the patient's home. Minor procedures such as removing fluid from the abdomen (on 60 occasions), or from the chest (12), and putting up an intra-venous drip for a short time to administer anti-tumour drugs (22) can all be done without the elaborate facilities of a hospital. For 20 of the patients with bowel impactions* we even gave a general anaesthetic to facilitate its removal. Only 82 had to be returned to hospital, so some 564 patients remained to die at home.

When admission to the hospice was necessary, it did not always have to be permanent. Thus 52 patients came in for a short stay to give the family a rest, to have diabetes or an infection controlled, or for intensive rehabilitation, and then returned home again.[238] Initially the Service was allotted 6 beds in the hospice, but this proved inadequate, as did 8. In order to have one bed empty most of the time, and to be able to admit patients for short rest periods, we have found that a domiciliary service of our size needs 12 beds, which means one in-patient bed for every six or seven patients at home. St Joseph's also has more than 40 other beds for people who could not go home to die. Thus over 60% of the hospice's dying patients are in their own homes at any one time.

Staffing

From the outset it was our diligent concern to establish a Service which could be copied in any big city if people willing to work hard enough would have a go. Joint finance and encouragement from the National Society for Cancer Relief (NSCR) and the City and East London Area Health Authority (AHA) made the development of the Service possible. The result is a pattern and precedent on which others can build.

In each of the Health Districts which we cover (see Figure A), one district nursing sister has specialized in care of the dying and joined the Macmillan team. The size

*Constipated motions blocking the lower bowel.

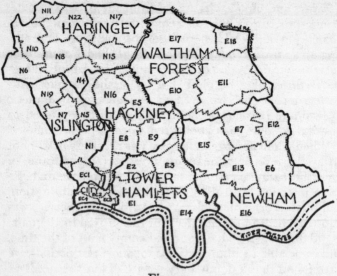

Figure A

of the team was dictated in part by the need to have enough staff to share the on-call rota for night duty, so that no one worked more than one night each week. The nurses obviously have to be district-nurse trained, and of considerable experience, stability and intelligence. There is no place in this work for people who 'become too involved', which, being interpreted, means people whose response to suffering in others is to feel sorry for themselves. The work is hard enough without having people in the team who need undue support themselves. Great comradeship will arise. Meetings will be numerous, the natural support they afford being sufficient. All meetings are directed to consideration of the patients or the work, not at some kind of therapy for the staff.

In any undertaking of this sort it is vital that all members of the team be able to work smoothly and happily together. Long hours and much sharing of work necessitate trust and friendship. New staff are chosen by a subcommittee of doctor, nurse and social worker, and are only offered a three-month contract. In view of the 1977 labour relations laws, this must be ruthlessly adhered to. In the three months every member of the team has to decide whether he can work with the applicant, as well as assessing the quality of his work and his willingness to work.

The Nurse's Work

Fifteen patients each is the comfortable maximum caseload that district nurses can handle in this kind of work, ideally paying 6–8 visits a day. This gives them time to reassess the patient's needs and therapy regularly, and to give that time to listening and conversing with the patient and his family which are so necessary in care of the dying. Even then she may well need to call on the other district nurses in her district to help with changing dressings, giving occasional injections, or doing time-consuming general nursing care. If any nurse's numbers push up towards 20 patients, the others in the team will have to go in to help her. Fortunately, so far, when one district is busy, another one has gone quiet. We dread the day when three or more districts become busy at once! By working as a team we have been able to absorb as many as 25 patients in one nurse's area because there is one nurse not attached to any district who helps out in the busiest locality.

These nurses have more responsibility and freedom than most district nurses. Discretion to alter therapy in response to the frequent changes in the patient's condition is allowed by the doctor. There is a limited range of drugs routinely prescribed which they can use at any time as the need arises. Mouth, bladder and bowel care are their total responsibility, no doctor's consent being needed for each enema or urinary catheter being used. They will carry out many routine pathological tests unprompted. Lack of freedom in these fields can paralyse district nurses at a time of urgent need, and deny relief to the patient for several days.

Our average patient receives 20 nurses' visits. At first, while he is mobile, they may be infrequent – say, once a week – but at the end, if coma has forced us to use injections, he may be seen every eight hours.

Each nurse is responsible to the community nursing officer in her district, meeting with her weekly. She has to contact any other district nurse already involved in any patient's care so that they can share out the work. There is certainly no attempt to push away any person whom the family is already finding supportive. Sharing the work is important because on any day the Macmillan nurse needs to know that she has enough time to sit down and converse with any patient who hints that he is wanting to talk.

The Doctor's Work

It has been found needful to have two doctors on duty every day in order to cope with our normal caseload of 70–85 patients. At night they are on call in case a crisis arises which the nurse on duty cannot manage alone. This means having three doctors – medical director, registrar and houseman – because a considerable teaching commitment also has to be met. The more senior doctor on duty sees any newly-referred patients, following up with a second visit the next day to see if his changes of therapy have in fact helped.

The first visit is a marathon and can easily take two hours. An exhaustive list of symptoms is checked off in problem-orientated colour-coded notes. Names and phone numbers of all persons who help to sustain the family are noted down. Social, nursing and medical needs have to be assessed and the patient thoroughly examined. Any laboratory tests or emergency treatments (e.g. urinary catheter) have to be instituted. And when the patient and doctor are both exhausted, there may begin another session with the relatives outside the front door. Whether or not the patient trusts the team will depend on his first

impressions during this visit. It helps if at least one troublesome symptom can be dramatically relieved within hours
– pain being the most amenable candidate. It will also be
necessary to establish in the family's mind a hierarchy of
responsibility. No patient is seen without the family
doctor's consent, and this is made clear at the door – 'Good
morning, Dr A. asked me to see Mrs B. about her pain.' A
brochure is given which explains that the Macmillan Service is always on call, in case the family doctor is ever
inaccessible. Patients are encouraged to keep hospital
appointments for as long as they are able,[239] and letters
about the patient's progress are sent frequently to all
doctors concerned.

More routine visits – conducted at the request of the
nurses – will be made by the junior doctor. Paging bleeps
are distributed among the team so that someone will be
somewhere near any emergency situation.

The Social Worker's Work

To win the family's trust by being a manipulator of welfare, and then to be the family's confidant and sustainer
as they are faced with death and bereavement, are roles
anyone in the team may have to fill, but which will be the
special concern of the social worker.

The main social problems which we encounter are
listed in Table 3. The most appropriate support in each
situation has to be found. What happens to the children if
the head of a one-parent family dies? How do you cope
with someone who is suicidal with grief? How can family
feuds exploding over a death-bed be handled? How can a
husband and wife be helped to communicate about their
plans for after the death of one of them? All such questions are regularly posed to a social worker in this field.
One or other member of the team was able to attend 151 of
the patients' funerals. This demonstrates our continued
concern to the family.

Once a month the Thursday staff meeting is devoted to

	NUMBER OF PATIENTS OUT OF 1,000
Caring relative coping alone	224
Caring relative also caring for young children	78
Caring relative also caring for an aged parent	22
Caring relative also caring for mentally ill person	18
Patient living alone	121
No relatives (or all contact broken off)	29
Second family bereavement in one year	17
Family rejecting patient	17
Family feuding: jealousies involving patient	12
Family hovering for money	5
Teenager was main caregiver	5

Table 3: Principal Social Problems Encountered

considering the needs of the bereaved. Most routine visits to families after a death will be paid by the nurses. But if a pathological grief reaction is anticipated (see Chapter 11) then the social worker will take over. Very seldom is it necessary to refer someone to a psychiatrist.

The social worker tries to meet every new patient to make her own assessment, but she does not get to the ones who are only in our care for a short time. So time-consuming is this part of the work that a welfare assistant or student is needed to free more of the social worker's time for work with the bereaved.

The Physiotherapist's Work

Maximizing mobility, helping to treat breathlessness,[181] and a certain amount of massage for bedbound patients are the preserve of the physiotherapist. In the last year she paid 434 visits to one quarter of the patients – which is more than four visits each. This contribution is a vital one. Doctors and nurses just do not have the training to be adequate substitutes.

Any patient whose chest infection is to be treated by antibiotics will be given postural drainage and breathing exercises.

A person who has been in bed for a long time may have got out of the habit of moving and walking. This immobility leads to the development of bedsores and stiffness. Over-protective relatives may unwittingly bring this upon a patient by doing too much for him, perhaps because they have been afraid to let him walk about. But there is no point in becoming bedbound before it is inevitable. A patient should walk as long as it pleases him to walk. It is better to get about leaning on a Zimmer walking frame than not to walk at all. If pain prevents him from being mobile, then once that has been removed he can be on his feet again provided he is given a little encouragement.[89] However, the patient should be warned to move cautiously. If the pain on movement was due to cancer weakening a bone, the pain was warning the patient that the bone was fragile. When the pain is taken away, if he is not careful he may do even more harm to the weakened bone.[114]

The dying may also have many other minor ailments besides their terminal one. These should not be neglected and allowed to cause discomfort. Such complaints as weak leg muscles, stiff neck, low back pain and stress incontinence (wetting a little on coughing) are often amenable to physiotherapy. Patients with pre-existent strokes and paralyses are also helped if their exercises are continued till the last possible day. An essential adjunct to this treatment is regular chiropody.

One of the principles of physiotherapy is setting the patient a goal. The skill in care of the dying is to set progressively lower goals, maintaining the patient's optimism but without offering false hopes. One may begin with active rehabilitation, progress to active exercises in bed, then passive movements, and finally massage.

All these efforts have to be coordinated by a secretarial paragon who answers the phone, types, advises, soothes. It helps if this person is a trained nurse who can give some advice to families on the phone. To receive calls at night we are bleeped by the local GP relief service. This ready availability at night has not been abused by patients.

The secretary, social worker, physiotherapist and a nurse are all paid by the NSCR.

Once a week there is a 'clinic'. All the patients who are well enough are brought by volunteers' cars to a social afternoon with tea and cakes and music. Seven or eight patients come each time, usually with a relative. One at a time they are seen in private by the doctor. For many patients who are otherwise housebound this is a welcome break, perhaps their only social life. It also gives an opportunity for those who may eventually need admission to the hospice to get to know it as a friendly place which they can trust. One patient attending our clinic told a nurse, 'I stayed in bed all day yesterday to be sure I would be strong enough for Dr Lamerton's party!' 262 patients were able to make 1,045 visits to the clinic in the three years.

This is hectic hard work. Some time has to be put aside to allow the mind to return to silence, and to reflect on the whole work. Each day after lunch a quiet time is put aside – at least half an hour – when anyone may sit and study, paint, meditate or whatever he will. Other breaks that have arisen spontaneously were a silent pause and scripture reading before the daily meeting at 8 a.m., and a weekly prayer meeting for any staff and their spouses who wish to attend.

Each year every member of the team is given a study week, over and above the normal holidays, when they usually go to share ideas with some other hospice group.

We have felt for some time that the keenest barometer of our team spirit and quality of care is the proportion of patients with whom a team member is present and watching at the actual moment of death. One or other member of the team was at the bedside of 83 of the patients at this crucial moment.

But in practical terms, just how successful were we? Table 4 shows our record in controlling a number of common troublesome symptoms. The total number of our patients suffering from the symptom is in the first column, and the percentage who were relieved totally of the symptom for most of the time that we knew them is then shown. By far the commonest reason for failure in controlling this kind of distress was in fact the patient's failure to take the drugs regularly. It seems there is a high price on total lack of self-discipline.*

	NUMBER OF PATIENTS WHO SUFFERED THIS SYMPTOM	PERCENTAGE WHO ENJOYED GOOD RELIEF OF SYMPTOM
Pain	750	92
Constipation	477	91
Vomiting	202	86
Nausea (without vomiting)	133	91
Loss of appetite	324	46
Diarrhoea	64	45
Cough	294	57
Breathlessness	289	36
Headache	58	91
Insomnia (not due to any other symptom)	69	77

Table 4: Success in Symptom Control

These are the successes. But failure does not mean the patient is tormented: we would offer sedation rather than allow that. It means the symptom was incompletely controlled and kept on coming back.

* All the figures would be even better in the controlled environment of the hospice itself – see pp. 26–7.

If those patients are excluded who were referred to us too late, so that we did not have time to tackle their symptoms, we have seen a steady improvement in our skill in controlling pain and in helping patients over mental distress:

	1975–6	1976–7	1977–8
Pain	88	90	95
Anxiety	36	46	46
Depression	43	44	47

Table 5: Percentage given good relief

Over the three years we have increased the number of patients' funerals we attend from one in ten to one in five. Although the average length of time a patient is in our care has remained much the same, the frequency of nursing visits has steadily increased. The proportion of patients first seen in the hospital before discharge home has increased from 3.4% to 7.8%. The number of patients introduced to us by a relative or friend who had heard of our reputation has also increased, as has the proportion referred by their family doctors (from 51% to 58%).

But in spite of some obvious strides forward, we become ever more aware of the magnitude of our task and our inadequacy for it. Staff meetings see much more soul-searching than back-patting. Criticism and suggestions for improvement are like fresh air, and much welcomed by the team.

Practical Points

So much for the hospice way. Now let us consider what can be done in any home given goodwill.[152]

Friends and neighbours often rally wonderfully to the aid of the dying. Perhaps the first thing to advocate is that the patient and his family should *accept* all the help offered. Refusal to do so is just a twisted form of not giving. With their help, it may be possible to arrange a night rota for attending to the patient's nocturnal needs.

Professor Wilkes found at least 13% of dying patients flatly refused to go into hospital.[413] They probably made the right choice. The prospect of caring for a dying relative or friend at home need not be overwhelming. In one study[414] a half of the patients died without ever needing difficult nursing care, and a further 20% were difficult to nurse for less than two weeks. In only 15% of the case histories examined did the period of difficulty last more than six weeks. This is the group who need specialized help. The same applies to children – there is no need at all to press for their admission to hospital at the end, provided they have adequate medical attention.

What is in fact expected of the doctor?

The patient's changing needs must be frequently assessed, but even if no alteration to his drugs is necessary, the doctor's visit is essential. Though the doctor may feel helpless his presence is reassuring.[3] Though he may not know what to say, the fact that he is there is comforting. His success in controlling symptoms and anticipating crises will ensure the patient's tranquil death and the family's sense of achievement. Thus the guilt so often experienced by the bereaved may be greatly softened or completely expiated through having successfully nursed a dying relative to the end. The sense of 'not having failed him' is a balm and a comfort to the grief-stricken family.[241]

The doctor should accept the patient's lead in whether they talk about his diagnosis. If the patient only wants reassurance, it still doesn't help for the doctor to lie.

In this way the dying patient and his family will start from a secure base of trust and understanding with their general practitioner. No unwanted knowledge will be given, nor any false hope of recovery. This is not to say that no hope at all is given; the hope is a sure one – 'I will always be available if you want me', and 'your symptoms will never be allowed to become unbearable'. It is a remarkable fact that, given those assurances, the patient will rarely abuse them. If he knows that

77

his questions will be given serious attention, he will ask only what he really wants to know. If he knows that he can get help when he is desperate he will not be phoning unnecessarily.[241]

One of the most embarrassing questions that a doctor gets asked is 'How long has he got?' There is just no way of knowing how long someone will live.[283] If he gives any more than a very approximate guess – 'could be two weeks, could be several months' – he is bluffing. Then when the patient doesn't die on the prescribed day or week, the doctor becomes mistrusted or an object of fun, and much frustrating distress is suffered by the relatives.

Drugs for the relief of symptoms will be prescribed by the family doctor. If the patient is needing a regular dose of a morphine mixture it will be necessary for the doctor to speak about it personally to the local chemist's shop. Pharmacists can be very destructive in how they label and hand over the mixtures, mainly out of ignorance. From red labels saying 'DANGEROUS DRUG' or even 'POISON' to dire warnings about addiction and overdose, or simply refusing to dispense it, they can alarm people quite unnecessarily (see Chapter 4). The doctor should see that the bottle is clearly labelled with what is in it (for the sake of any other doctor attending the patient), which means initialling the N.P. box at the top of the prescription form. And incidentally, every patient dying of cancer is entitled to free National Health prescriptions under the 'continuing disability' heading.

Since much of the patient's comfort depends on taking drugs regularly and reliably, the doctor should keep them to the minimum and make sure the family have a clear timetable. Table 6 shows the kind of drug schedule which the Macmillan Service patients receive.

When, towards the end, the patient is almost comatose, there are two main indications for calling the doctor: if the patient's breathing becomes rattly, or if he gets very restless. In both cases an injection may be needed. Of course if a nurse is present with the patient the doctor

TIME	NAME OF DRUG	DESCRIPTION OF DRUG	DOSE
7am.	MACMILLAN MIXTURE	Brown medicine for pain	One Blue Spoon
	PREDNISOLONE	Red tablet for appetite	1 Tablet
11am	MACMILLAN MIXTURE		One Blue Spoon
	MODURETIC	Diamond-shaped tablet for swollen ankles	1 Tablet
3pm	MACMILLAN MIXTURE		One Blue Spoon
	PREDNISOLONE		1 Tablet
7pm	MACMILLAN MIXTURE		One Blue Spoon
	DORBANEX FORTE	Orange medicine to keep the bowels regular	One Blue Spoon
11pm	MACMILLAN MIXTURE		One Blue Spoon
	PREDNISOLONE		1 Tablet

NAME Mrs. A. PATIENT   DATE 29·3·81

Please bring this card with you to every clinic at St. Joseph's Hospice

Table 6

with foresight can arrange to leave the injections ready at the bedside in case they are needed.

The 'death rattle' is partly due to saliva trickling into the patient's windpipe when he is too weak to cough it up, and partly to waterlogging of the lungs as the heart fails. An injection of atropine can help, and so can correct positioning of the patient. He should be placed on his side, with his head quite low. A pillow behind his back will prevent him rolling on to his back again, and the position is held by crossing the uppermost arm and leg

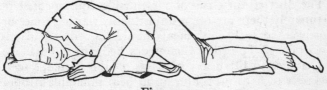

Figure B

across the body – see Figure B. On the other hand some patients breathe more easily if they are sitting up – this would particularly apply to a person who was more alert. In this case there is the constant nuisance of him slipping down flat. A 'bed donkey' is designed to overcome this. It is made by rolling a large pillow in a sheet to make a sausage. It is put at the bottom of the bed for his feet to rest on, and held in place by tucking in the two ends of the sheet on either side of the bed.

When a patient is restless, one should first check that it is not due to a distended bladder or packed bowels. If he has not passed urine for a day or more, the nurse or doctor could try inserting a catheter: they may get a 2-litre surprise. But the failing lungs and heart may be simply not supplying the brain with enough oxygen, and this can be a cause of restlessness. Giving oxygen does not help. The patient at this stage just needs very heavy sedation: perhaps three or four times the dose of sedative drugs usually used. We find that the best drug for this purpose is methotrimeprazine (Veractil or Nozinan).* If there is any likelihood that the patient has any pain, an analgesic should be added to the injection. At this stage we use either Temgesic 0.6 mg 12-hourly for moderate pain – or methadone for severe pain. Methadone should only be used at the very end of someone's life because if used for more than a few days it can be dangerously cumulative. Its advantage is that it lasts for eight hours, so only three injections a day are needed. (See p. 50.)

If the doctors or nurses are perplexed at any time, they can always telephone for advice to St Christopher's Hospice in London: 01-778 9252.

The district nurse can obtain nursing equipment. Unfortunately there are often unjustifiable waiting times or shortages, so such equipment should be ordered in advance of need if possible. Commodes, bedpans and urinals; bed cradles to lift heavy blankets off the patient's feet; backrests to help prop him up in bed; inflatable rubber rings for him to sit on if loss of weight has made his bottom bony; spouted feeding cups, drawsheets and incontinence pads can all be lent by the nursing service. The supply of wheelchairs is so inefficiently handled that

* If this fails, our second choice is IM phenobarbitone 200–400 mg.

it is unlikely that one will be available at just the time when the patient may need one. The dying need equipment quickly, which is not one of the Health Service's strong points. (In the USA the American Cancer Society also lends food liquidizers, an example which the Macmillan Service has followed.)[22]

One of the main concerns of the district nurse will be care of the patient's pressure areas (over the sacrum and coccyx at the base of the spine, the heels and the hips) to try to prevent bedsores. This is usually possible, though not always. For a patient who is not incontinent and is still slightly mobile, the nurse may be able to provide a sheepskin to sit on. For someone bedbound and not moving much, a ripple bed will help. This is plastic with inflatable ribs which alternately fill and empty so that the patient's weight is taken by different areas. The pump for it has to be set correctly for the patient's weight. But this equipment is no substitute for regular attention to the pressure areas, about which a nurse can teach the family. Ideally, if the skin looks as if it might break, the patient should be turned two-hourly and the areas massaged gently with a barrier cream such as Conotrane. If the skin is already broken, the area all round it is massaged. If it is a painful superficial sore it can be eased by a local anaesthetic application (e.g antiseptic lignocaine urethral gel). If infection of the sore is troublesome, honey is a good disinfectant to put on the dressing. If a deep hole develops, slough should be removed and the cavity cleaned with hydrogen peroxide ten volumes solution, which produces an oxygen-rich foam, killing gangrene germs. (Care should be taken not to splash this solution in the eyes.) Deep bedsores can be packed with sterile gauze after the hole has been sprayed with a disinfectant – Cicatrin powder or Disadine spray will suffice. Many other forms of treatment are favoured in different hospitals, but this one can be carried out at home.

The two-hourly turning will have to be compromised a little at night – ensure that there are no wrinkles in the sheets under the patient before settling him. To turn someone requires almost no effort if you use the arm and bent leg as levers to swing his shoulders and pelvis over. The district nurse can demonstrate this, as well as easy techniques for lifting someone up the bed or out of it on to the commode. The important thing to watch is that the pressure areas are not rubbed against the sheet as a patient is moved.

Moving an unconscious or semi-conscious person who cannot cooperate is a job for two people, one on each side, linking their hands under him and coordinating their efforts by saying 'one, two, three, lift'. When the balance and position are exactly right, even heavy people are easy to move provided the manoeuvre is not rushed. Full attention is required, so social conversation at the time should be avoided.

Another much-dreaded problem – which is a bit of a bogeyman really – is incontinence. It is just not necessary nowadays. If the bladder muscle is not functioning properly, a physiotherapist may be able to strengthen it with a Faradic stimulator, or the doctor may give Cetiprin tablets to relax it. If this doesn't work, the men can be fitted with a Uridom. The urine goes into a bag down a tube which is held on by a condom. This can be glued to the penis with Warne Skin Adhesive. (Put the adhesive *round* the penis, not in strips along it, to avoid leaks.) If a Uridom is unsuccessful, and in female patients, there should be no hesitation about inserting a catheter. This is a tube which is pushed into the bladder. It cannot drop out because a little balloon holds it in. Infection of a catheter can be prevented by a once-weekly dose of a long-acting sulphonamide tablet or some similar drug. If he is still mobile the patient could have the urine bag strapped to his leg, suspended from his pyjama cord under the dressing gown or, for the ladies, carried in a little crocheted handbag. Catheters have to be changed periodically. Lots of rules are made about this, but in practical fact they are usually changed when they become blocked

– which is betrayed by urine leaking round the tube instead of down it. Only 7.4% of our 1,000 patients were incontinent of urine. At some stage in their illness we catheterized 220 of them.

Incontinence of the bowels is treated by preventing it. The patient is given codeine to make him slightly constipated. Then, when convenient, he sits on the commode after two Dulcolax suppositories have been inserted. Thus he only has his bowels open when he wants to. (But beware, a common cause of soiling is 'spurious diarrhoea' due to leakage past a bowel impaction.)

The nurses will no longer be worried by temperature and pulse measurements – for which there is no point in disturbing him – but they should check the mouth for thrush at every visit, and the bowels for constipation. No fewer than 48% of our 1,000 patients were constipated badly enough for it to be causing them unpleasant symptoms when they were first referred to us. Of these, there were 90 with impactions in the rectum (see Chapter 4).

Adequate care of the mouth is essential. It pays to have ill-fitting dentures refashioned as long as the person can eat. Chewing gum may freshen up the mouth and help the patient to make saliva. Thrush looks like flecks of milk curd stuck to the gums and palate, each surrounded by a red inflamed flare. It is a constant nuisance to debilitated patients, especially if they have been given an antibiotic. It can be very uncomfortable but is easy to treat with Nystan mouth drops every four hours. The Nystan should also be put in the water in which any false teeth are stored at night.

When a patient becomes very weak the mouth may be gently cleaned with Smith & Nephew foam-stick applicators.[66] The mouth may drop open and become dry. Water should be given in frequent small quantities as long as the person can swallow. A medicine dropper helps to measure it into his mouth. A gauze wick with one end in ice water and the other in the mouth for the patient to suck has been recommended. Ice wrapped in gauze may be placed inside the cheek to melt gradually, replacing saliva. On the other hand if there is too much saliva, it may be absorbed by wads of gauze placed between the cheek and gums. The patient should be lying on his side so that the fluid doesn't trickle down his windpipe, making him cough.

For a patient who is seriously dehydrated, causing him discomfort from dry mouth and thirst, a rectal infusion of tap water may occasionally be tried. A litre can be given over 6–8 hours, dripping from an intravenous giving set down into a soft rubber tube inserted through the anus for 30 cm. If this is running smoothly, the district nurse can leave it and come back later, or even let it drip overnight while the patient sleeps.

Sometimes a cancer can break down a patch of skin producing an ulcer. If this gets deep it may be helped by radiotherapy, but often cannot be. Infection may develop and the result be a smelly discharge. We tackle these by cleaning with hydrogen peroxide (p. 81) and then putting in live yogurt. This produces an acid environment which most germs dislike, and prevents colonization from any other germs by the growth of its own lactobacilli over all surfaces. This is a harmless bacillus which does not invade the body cells, so causes no inflammation.

If she needs help, the district nurse can also call upon the domiciliary chiropody service.

She may be able to get a night nurse to sit with a very weak patient so that his family can get some rest at least one or two nights a week. However, such nurses and the funds for them are hard to come by in some areas.[267]

There are many ways a social worker's help may be needed. Financial problems may be an embarrassment: special food for invalids is expensive, nursing aids have to be bought, heating costs will go up, and all at a time when family income has dropped because the patient's or the nursing relative's income has stopped. The social worker can steer them through the jungle of forms for claiming Supplementary Benefits, rent rebates, income tax relief and Attendance Allowance. Under special circumstances an Invalid Care Grant may be claimed. The National Society for Cancer Relief also gives grants to help with all kinds of difficulties and expenses. Most of these involve some kind of means test. The Attendance Allowance is substantial, but only available after a patient has required attention for six months. It is applied for on a form from the Post Office or the DHSS in the fifth month.

Local Social Services Departments can provide home helps and meals-on-wheels. The former are often in short supply, and the latter may not be provided at weekends. If someone is likely to be dying at home, it is a great advantage to have a telephone. The social worker should explore ways that one might be financed.

Sometimes a patient or a spouse struggling on alone may be too proud to ask the rest of the family for help, but wouldn't mind the social worker putting in a word. Indeed, all concerned may be glad of someone to talk to. So many problems may come to light. There may be quite groundless fears that cancer is dirty, infectious or contagious, needlessly putting up barriers between people.[28] If branches of the family who have previously quarrelled are called in, they may find themselves facing one another across the bed. One has 'done more for Mum' than the other, so one is feeling guilty and the other resentful. If they are already communicating with a trained mediator like a social worker, major feuds can be averted.[300]

There is much that friends and neighbours can do. Their visits may be tiring for the patient, so need to be short, but they are nevertheless needed. Television alone is certainly not a remedy for boredom. What will the patient do with his hands? Is there someone who will play cards, buy in supplies for a sedentary hobby, or even take him out for a while? The patient should not be all alone when he eats if possible. A small table might be squeezed into the bedroom so someone else can come and eat with him.

Just because someone is an invalid, they need not be regarded as useless. The ladies can still plan meals and draw up shopping lists, control the housekeeping funds, and supervise children for as long as possible. The man should still be consulted as master of the house. Dignity should be preserved with regular shaving and hairdressing. So that the ill person can continue to be in the centre of the family life, it is often a good idea to bring his bed into the living room. If that is not possible, then at least he needs an easily accessible bell to hail people with (provided this summons does not become a tyranny!).

If the patient's appetite is failing, and doesn't respond to such medical measures as tonics or prednisolone tablets (5 mg three times daily – raises metabolic rate and counters raised blood calcium),[399] then he needs to be reassured and given only small portions and variety. Fresh fruit and eggs should be high priorities. If the patient cannot take much sustenance, Complan contains all the vitamins and other nutrients that the patient needs. It is less sickly if made up with water rather than milk. When a dying person is very weak there is certainly no need to push food into him if he just doesn't want it. But Complan can spoil the appetite, so should only be given to someone already not eating. There is no reason why people who are dying should not enjoy alcohol, especially at night when it can be more use than sleeping tablets.

To prevent a cancer in the gullet from blocking it completely, surgeons sometimes insert a tube to provide a way through (Mousseau-Barbin, Souttar's or Celestin's tubes). These should be regularly disinfected by giving the patient runny honey after meals. Avoid lumps of meat, cabbage and green salad which may readily block the tube. But if it does block and the patient feels food is stuck in his gullet, or regurgitates some of it, drinking a quick swig of fizzy lemonade usually clears it.

Should the patient have to be fed by someone else this can be done beautifully or very badly. Remember the patient's favourite tit-bits may still be appreciated (jellied eels for Cockneys, black pudding in Leeds, haggis in Glasgow, udders and tripe in Manchester. Ugh!) Don't ram the food in. Here is an excellent explanation by a girl who was almost totally paralysed by motor neurone disease. She dictated this article to a nurse by blinking in Morse code, because she was too weak to speak:

Possibly I am particularly sensitive, but I hate to be fed. Nevertheless it makes an enormous difference to one's enjoyment of a meal if the person helping takes a real interest in what she is doing. I know that it must require infinite patience, but there are some people who will go to endless trouble to keep the food hot, and make it as tasty as possible. They also give the impression that there is nothing they would rather be doing at that particular time. Others, however, will carry on an animated conversation with another, whilst holding an appetizing forkful – just out of reach! – or stare out of the window, in deep thought, while one watches the food getting cold.

The person in whom I have most confidence is the one who goes about her work slowly and deliberately, telling what she is about to do, giving me the opportunity to indicate if anything is wrong. She seems to get through her work just as quickly as the one who exercises a more forceful approach.

The rest of this essay is equally valuable reading, particularly for nurses or physiotherapists.[257]

Another service which may be needed from relatives is tending a colostomy (where the bowel is brought to the front of the abdomen because of obstruction in the back passage). There are many different types of bag or appliance and the patient himself, before he is too weak, will be the best instructor as to how to change his particular colostomy. Usually it is a simple procedure – it will need cleaning with ordinary warm water. Plaster marks may be removed using solvent ether. If the skin round the colostomy should become sore, patches of Stomahesive placed under the appliance are often very effective. The Colostomy Welfare Group* may be able to help with problems, or the district nursing sister who visits might ask a specialist nurse to give further advice. Generally colostomies, once established, are relatively easy to care for.

If there is an odour from the colostomy or from an ulcer, a deodorant solution like Nilodor can be put – one or two drops – on the dressing or in the bag. If there is difficulty in disposing of soiled dressings they should at least be put in sealed plastic bags. Should there be enormous quantities to throw away, the district nurse can ask the Environmental Health Officer at the Town Hall to have them collected.

There can be problems for everyone if a cancer spreads to the brain. In fact this often happens without giving the patient any symptoms at all. A host of different patterns of illness can present, but often there will be one-sided weakness, like a stroke. The patient may have double vision, and is likely to get headaches and nausea and a few have fits. If the cancer does not respond to anti-tumour drugs or radiotherapy, there may be nothing to do but give anti-nausea drugs and something to prevent fits. Occasionally a steroid drug might give the patient a brief respite of borrowed time. When this works, he is so improved at first that he may be lulled into hoping for a cure. The temporary nature of this treatment must be stressed – at least to close relatives, because later it will have to be discontinued again (p. 54). These times can be very hard because the patient may undergo personality changes which make him hard to meet for anyone but the most adoring and close. More than one in ten of our 1,000 patients had problems from brain involvement, which gives some idea of the commonness of this complication.

When nursing a semi-conscious or apparently comatose patient, always remember that they may still be able to hear acutely even if they cannot respond. Careless comments over unconscious patients are heard more often

* Colostomy Welfare Group, 38 Eccleston Square, London SW1 (01-828 5175).

than one would think. Such a patient may also still be able to feel pain, which is why pain-killing injections will be continued even to a comatose patient within hours of his death. They are to relieve pain, and are not going to shorten his life.

If someone's death is easy and peaceful with no complications at all – as is usually the case – there may be nothing much for the family to do. There is then a tendency to hover anxiously and look for some activity. But it is more important for the patient that they are simply present, with him, than anything they can do. No one should die alone. Holding his hand may be all that is needed.

As soon as someone in the family is dying, the relatives will start to hear fantastic stories. 'Cancer blocking the bowels, eh? Ooh yes, Mrs Smith's brother's friend's niece had that – due to phlebitis of the caruminous glands or something – and she took olive oil and camomile tea with pepper in it. Done her the world of good. Doctor said it was a miracle.' Or worse, there may be tales of magic cures at great expense in Bavaria or Mexico or Antarctica, tempting the family to bankrupt themselves, and causing the patient exhausting and unnecessary journeys. Faith healers have generally done good for our patients (though never cured one of his cancer) but relatives should be suspicious of those who charge a lot. Families should always seek the opinion of a doctor they trust before embarking on treatments from charlatans and quacks which may do more harm than good. Several of our patients have had nasty experiences with these, normally well-meaning, characters.

Should there be questions of any kind about the care of patients with cancer, anyone may ring the Information Bureau at the Marie Curie Foundation for individual advice – 01-730 9157.

Neighbourly assistance, perhaps organized by the vicar, can help to shore up a family at this time. Obviously they would be embarrassed to ask for help themselves. If a neighbour has a car, can they take the patient to his hospital out-patients appointment? Ambulances so often come at the wrong time, take ages for the journey and bounce the patient around. (Indeed, a domiciliary visit by the hospital consultant in company with the family doctor may often be more appropriate.) Neighbours can offer the use of their phone – night or day. They can pop in to help lift a patient or to do the shopping. Sometimes it is kinder to let the patient's own spouse have a break and go shopping by staying with him for a while.

When the patient dies he will stop breathing and gradually become pale and cold, all peacefully. It is enough to remove excess bedding, leaving just one pillow, and to lie him straight. The undertaker will wash him down. The mouth is held closed – by a book or similar-shaped object (e.g. a Kleenex box) – under the chin. The eyelids are closed. Heating in the room should be turned off. The first person needed is the doctor, who will write a death certificate (see p. 133). As soon as that is done the undertaker can be contacted. The skill and tact of most of these gentlemen constitutes the best possible grief therapy. They guide relatives over any complications during early bereavement. It helps the doctor and undertaker if they can be informed as soon as possible whether a burial or a cremation will be required, since the latter involves the doctor in filling in forms. As soon as the death certificate is written, the undertaker can remove the body (unless the family prefer it to remain in a cool room at home). Before he does this it is usually best to take children of the family in to say goodbye unless they are horrified by the idea. Let them look at the body, and touch it if they wish, but hold their hand.

All sorts of frills can make a funeral more expensive. Embalming is unnecessary and only preserves the body for a very short time. Burial is a costly affair, especially if fancy caskets, brick-lined graves and carved marble headstones are used. Sometimes families feel they should do the best by a dead person, and waste a lot of money.

The best should be done before the person dies, then there is no need to compensate afterwards with an ostentatious funeral.

Once arrangements with the undertaker have been made the death has to be registered at the local registry office of births, marriages and deaths. That means taking the deceased person's medical card with the death certificate to the Registrar during the rather short hours that he is available (ask the undertaker when these are). There is a 'death grant' of £30 to offset the cost of the funeral which the Registrar will invite the family to claim. He will want to know how many life insurance policies the deceased had, since a copy of the death certificate will have to be purchased for each company.

If the deceased had written a will, ask his solicitor about it.

Conclusion

The last word in this chapter shall go to Barbara McNulty,[240] who pioneered this field of home care for the dying, speaking of her first three years' experience of going out into the community from St Christopher's Hospice.

To sum up, I would like to suggest that the care of the dying is a specialist concern, and that this is not sufficiently recognized. A person should be able to die at home if he wishes. He should have easy access to a specialist unit bed with the possibility of discharge home and continuity of care.

Financial aid should be given to those families who wish to care for a patient at home, and in realistic proportion to what they are saving the State in hospital expenses; and such aid should be available easily and quickly.

It is self-evident that support at home should include not only the improvement in continuity of medical care, increased night nursing facilities, realistic financial help, but also the immediate availability of relevant aids, and all this must be given with an understanding of the urgency, because there is so little time.

Better liaison between hospital and community is very much part of our present thinking. The experiment in which I have participated during these past three years has shown how close this liaison can be, how greatly the patient benefits from such a liaison and what satisfaction it can bring to all participants.

The value of this liaison service between the hospice and the community can be gauged first by the welcome and relief expressed by patients and their families; they frequently say, 'I feel so much safer now. I feel I am not alone now.'

6. Dying in Hospital

✤

Some 66 of our 1,000 home care patients were first seen in the ward of a referring hospital. Since their physical distress – in terms of pain, constipation and other symptoms – was little different from that suffered by patients whom we first saw at home, one must question the value of admitting dying patients to hospital. In 1965 the Registrar General's statistics for England and Wales showed that 38% of all deaths occurred at home. By 1975 the figure was little over 30%.[396] Is this trend justified?[119]

People may die in hospital from many different diseases[111] – pneumonia or severe bronchitis, heart attacks, heart failure, strokes, thrombosis and gangrene; cancers and leukaemias; tremors and paralyses, arthritis and fractures. Whatever the nature of the illness, there are certain principles to be observed. Before it becomes apparent that the disease is incurable, most of these patients will have undergone some attempt at curative treatment. But once this is abandoned, it will give place to symptomatic treatment. This will involve the whole hospital staff in a complete change of approach.[441] The different concept of 'Care of the Dying' will govern their actions when a 'trial of therapy' has failed (p. 126).

Symptomatic Treatment

When cure is no longer the aim, the staff will use all their skill to bring the patient comfort, treating each symptom as it arises. Many doctors and nurses find this adjustment in aim difficult.[345] A new restraint is now needed in the use of drugs and other life-saving measures.[234] The correct treatment of pneumonia is a case in point.

In the elderly and infirm, bronchopneumonia is not the violent disease with high fever and shortness of breath which we see in a young person. Instead, without causing much distress, it gently induces drowsiness and a peaceful death. The onset of pneumonia is an indication that the patient's body has stopped fighting, and that he is ready to go. Sometimes – by no means always – the patient's condition can be temporarily improved by giving him oxygen, antibiotics, physiotherapy, vitamins and perhaps blood transfusions. The apparent success of this treatment might give the staff a glowing sense of achievement, so there is a great temptation to have a try. But if a man has a cancer which is spreading, or if he is already paralysed and senile from a severe stroke, such interference would be inappropriate, bad, 'meddlesome medicine'. In these circumstances, the correct treatment for bronchopneumonia is to give the patient an opiate, which suppresses breathlessness and any pain, steroid drugs which relieve the fever and some of the weariness and loss of appetite, and, at the end, a belladonna drug can be added to the narcotic to dry up the secretions in the throat and lungs, with a tranquillizer to ease any feelings of panic. Covering the patient's face with an oxygen mask does not usually make much difference to his breathing, but can worsen his feeling of suffocation, and is a subtle way of avoiding communication with him. The aim, after all, is to ease the breathlessness, not to produce better blood-gas results.

There are some infections which cause such discomfort that their treatment with antibiotics is expedient, though only for purposes of relief, not of healing. Infections of the bladder, mouth and eyes, and of bedsores are examples. It is not necessary to use drip-feeding into veins, operations like a gastrostomy (a tube direct into the stomach because the gullet is blocked), which merely lengthen the process of dying, or experimental new drugs which have been eagerly advertised.

The doctor has to realign his whole attitude to his patient. First of all he must discover which symptom distresses the patient most. This can be quite a surprise. Constipation may be causing him more concern than his cancer of the face; having a dry mouth may be more burdensome than a growth the size of a football. If pain is present, then drugs must be given in sufficient quantity to control it (p. 48), and they should be given immediately the patient is admitted to the hospital. This gives him a sense of security from the outset. At all times there must be a pause before active therapy is begun and the question asked: is it really relevant at this time for this patient?

The most drastic test of this rational approach comes on the RARE occasions when a patient's cancer bleeds profusely and fatally. All one's training and instinct cry for frantic action. Stop the haemorrhage! There is an urge to rush about and do things. But remembering that, even if it can be stopped now, it will only bleed again and kill him later, one can see that the patient just needs someone to hold on to.[107] Several hospitals keep a large red blanket in a handy cupboard for such occasions. This can soak up the blood without making it obvious, so that the patient is spared the frightening sight of spreading redness. Curtains are quickly pulled round the bed, and someone must sit on the bed as a companion for the person.

Likewise, when a total bowel obstruction develops in a patient with widespread abdominal cancer, and the surgeon cannot operate further, this should be seen as a terminal event. Anti-spasmodics like propantheline (Pro-Banthine) combined with sedation with chlorpromazine (Largactil) are much kinder at this stage than 'drip and suck' treatment which merely ensures that the patient takes three weeks to die instead of three days. Sometimes bowel blockage produces distension. The doctor can deflate this, for a dying patient, by puncturing the distended loop of bowel, through the skin, with a large hypodermic needle and letting out the gas. The procedure is painless.

The Patient is a Person

One discipline worth observing in a hospital is never to write a patient's name – even when filling in X-ray forms or writing a private note on the back of the hand – without Mr, Mrs or Miss in front of it. Otherwise we mentally demote the person, and this attitude shows in all our actions.

Hospital administration can too easily lose sight of the needs of a patient. In one I saw a big graph on the wall comparing different surgeons' statistics of 'patient throughput'. Empty beds and beds occupied for more than a week by one patient were marked in red, bringing opprobrium on the surgeon concerned, irrespective of the standard of his medicine. Perhaps doctors intent on promotion may think in terms of 'cases'. The acute ones may be considered more interesting because they are more taxing on the memory and intellect, and may fill a niche in the hunt for more diverse experience. Being usually overworked, nurses can narrow down the sphere of interest they take in the patients, and may answer the question 'Which is Mrs Henderson?' with 'She's the breast in bed twenty-two.' A 'good patient' is one who never complains and quietly fits into the system without question. It follows that a frightened patient who asks questions, or a dignified one who wishes to go on being Mrs Henderson, will be a nuisance, a 'bad patient'.

Of course these mistakes are not made everywhere. When they are, it is pointless to criticize the hospital staff for treating people as less than men, when their emotions are just a reflection of values throughout society. In spite of the strains under which doctors and nurses generally find themselves, however, the special circumstances of dying patients should always call forth respect.

The patient will probably have a suspicion of his diagnosis. Members of the staff may have let hints slip from their lips or actions and his suspicions and fears can be dreadful. In these circumstances it is essential that he clearly understands who has ultimate responsibility for his case, and that that person spends some time with him.[423] Since there is always something to be done for a patient, it is inexcusable to by-pass his bed on ward rounds even if he is, or seems to be, asleep. Palliative surgery would have to be suggested with utmost discretion and gentleness if it is not to be refused point blank.[123] Even more tact is needed if the patient is sent to die at home or in a hospice when the hospital has no more to offer him and the bed is needed urgently. The significance of the move will probably be obvious, and not helped by sugar-coated lies about 'going for convalescence'. In the long term his failure to recover will be easier for the patient to bear if he has been warned that he will need nursing care for longer than it can be given in a busy general ward.[330]

The patient should never be made to feel rejected, useless or in the way.[227] He may be greatly helped by his fellow patients, and may in turn support others, by helping them to cope with problems he has already faced.[432] Frequent and, if possible, regular visits from family and friends will be the mainstay of his morale. If they find the visiting painful or embarrassing, it may help for them to be joined for a while by someone less involved, perhaps a nurse, a social worker or a responsible volunteer. The best catalyst of all for facilitating warm interaction between people is the family's new baby. Children should never be excluded from the hospital for fear of frightening them. They can make visiting so much easier, and bring the dying patient an assurance of new life and continuity. It has been our experience that they are not distressed themselves.

Many patients with terminal illnesses cannot be discharged from hospital for one reason or another. In Dr Exton–Smith's series[111] some 60% of the patients were already bedridden before admission. The longer a patient is in the ward, the less attention he tends to receive from the doctors. The nursing may be heavy, which takes valuable staff away from acutely ill patients. This process was called in the *Lancet* a 'blocked bed'.[207]

It is easy for a patient to be regarded as socially dead before he is actually dead. The nurses often ritually acknowledge this by pulling the covers higher and higher, obscuring more and more of the patient (yet the ward temperature never changed!). The physiotherapist and occupational therapist have much to contribute to terminal care. They should be involved early in the patient's admission and continue to visit – if only socially – to the end. The dietitian and chiropodist can also help his well-being. The chaplain will usually have a helpful contribution to make: without him as a member of the caring team, the care is incomplete. Doctor, priest and nurse should collaborate around the bed of a dying patient.[127]

Should the patient be able to go home, he will need an ample supply of drugs with simple instructions as to what to take and when. The GP will urgently need – preferably by phone, if only to his receptionist – not only details of drugs and diagnosis, but also a briefing on exactly what the patient and his family have been told about his illness.[57]

The Family in the Hospital

The death of a person should leave his family with no regrettable memories.

They should be involved in his care as surely as they would be if he were at home. They can help the nurses with feeding him, turning him, washing him and so on. As this is their last offering to him, they want to be as intimately close to him as possible. Think of the person you most love, and then imagine having to say goodbye from a distance.[354]

If visiting is proving too expensive for the family, the

social worker may be able to get money to help with fares from such charities as the National Society for Cancer Relief.* She can also help them with their feelings of guilt at having failed to go on caring for the patient at home. If he returns to their care for a while, the hospital consultant's continued interest can be confirmed by visits from the social worker. She can help to arrange hospice admission or convalescence, as well as informing the consultant when the patient needs readmission if the family are having difficulties. Often a patient will not accept his invalid state until he has tried a period at home and found for himself that he cannot manage. For cancer patients who need heavy nursing it may be possible to secure a holiday in the nearest Marie Curie Home, to give the relatives a rest. Margaret Bailey recommends a holiday together for the whole family while the patient is still strong enough.[19]

The social worker has to resist the temptation to avoid the patient by concentrating on helping the relatives. In a hospital she may be the only person with the time to sit and listen to him, and as she is the 'lay' member of the team, some patients may find it easier to talk to her than to the doctors or the nurses.

These families will take priority on the services of the social worker because of the short time limit involved. Often her prime duty will be to help them to face up to their imminent bereavement, and later they may need help with handling funerals, estates, and grief.

While the patient is in hospital, someone will have to keep the relatives informed of his progress and expectations. This task is commonly delegated to the houseman or ward sister and can be difficult because the hospital staff do not usually know the family very well. If no real relationship has been established, it is always worth considering whether the family doctor is not a much better person to break hard news to the family, particularly as he is then available for follow-up. The best use can be

* 30 Dorset Square, London NW1 (01-402 8125).

made of this relationship if the doctor has his own beds in a local cottage hospital.[205]

News of the imminent death of a patient can be as hard for his relatives to accept as it is for the patient himself. I was recently asked by Mrs H., whose husband had bowel cancer, 'There isn't anything to worry about is there Doctor?' I decided to break the news to them gently, in stages, and parried the question by saying, 'Not really, but of course the colostomy will be permanent now.' The next time I saw her I told her that he would have the fluid drawn off from his tummy frequently for quite a long time 'because the irritation is still there'. With each new piece of information she expressed surprise and consternation. Then my partner returned from holiday and told me he had already taken Mrs H. through this process once, and had told her this diagnosis before going on holiday!

Little of the first interview will be assimilated. A common reaction is to plead that the patient should not be told. But more than once I have been asked by a patient not to distress his wife with such news, while at the same time the wife has been asking me to conceal the diagnosis from her husband. If the situation where only one of a couple has been informed should arise, then the other may later ask what the doctor said. I have helped several people in this predicament by returning with them to the patient's bed and saying something like 'Hello, Mr Heath, your wife has just been helping me to fill up your forms, and she tells me you are interested in sailing ...' etc. This avoids a clash of opinions in the first meeting, and defers difficult conversations to a less fraught later time.

When the patient does die, his family may again find the fact hard to accept. It helps if they can have been present and seen that the end was peaceful. Dr Cicely Saunders points out that to have said goodbye can be a great consolation, especially if it can be said that 'Last time he woke up, you were the last person he saw.'

The family can be asked if the patient would have liked

to give the corneas of his eyes for a surgeon to graft on to someone else. Only a doctor or nurse who has become a friend of the family, and who was seen to give tender caring to the patient before he died, is in a position to make this request, however. Relatives should be reassured that this will not disfigure the body. Neither this nor a post-mortem should be requested lightly by someone who has not earned the family's respect. If other organs are wanted for transplanting, then it is the consultant's duty to ask for them. To deal with this particular exigency, ethical codes are being developed in all countries to ensure that the patient's death is confirmed by an independent doctor not associated with the transplanting surgeon. The request for a post-mortem examination often shocks a family, so it needs to be done with great tact.[274] We are still awfully ignorant of how cancer spreads and how our treatments affect the body. Autopsies in great numbers are essential if we are to learn.

Even if a body is dead, it is still the most magnificent set of tools yet to have arisen on this earth. And this is not the only reason why it is worthy of respect, for it is still the symbol of a man. His loved ones will refer to it as if it were still the person. When the idea of a post-mortem examination is mentioned by the doctor, his request is often met with a look of anguish and a question such as 'Does that mean they'll cut him open?' 'Haven't they messed him about enough?' or 'Please let him rest now: I don't want that.'

Whatever we do outwardly, it is the *inner* respect that matters. I asked a nurse to tell me about the last washing of a body, and what she wrote shows this respect very clearly:

To nurse the dying was for me one of the most rewarding types of nursing. I was afraid of death when I first began and therefore chose to do orthopaedic nursing to avoid meeting it. In my general training hospital we were gently introduced to death. If a patient died, an experienced senior nurse would take a junior and teach her very gently how to do the last wash. The atmosphere of the room, the beauty of the ritual and reverence of the washing and the Presence in the room, removed from me this fear of death.

The last wash was done in two parts, and between the two parts the priest came and said some prayers. At first when I became attached to a patient who was dying, I did not want to be there to see him die or to perform the last wash, but later it was the opposite. To be able to perform that last act of service was important to me and when I became the senior nurse I was very careful to be gentle with the new junior who was meeting death for the first time.

Finally the hospital staff should mobilize community services for the after-care of the relatives, a duty which often goes by default. When someone dies in hospital his family doctor in particular should be informed the same day. The ward staff themselves may be able to help some bereaved relatives by inviting them to come back to give voluntary help.[305] Often they have been visiting for some considerable time, have proved themselves helpful, and know the ward routine and most of the other patients. This protects them from too drastic a change of habits when they have been coming daily to the hospital for months.

Some Recent Approaches

While every community of between a quarter and a half million people needs its hospice, some hospitals have exerted themselves to improve their own care of the dying by establishing special teams or units. In Montreal,[260] the Palliative Care Unit of the Royal Victoria Hospital is one approach involving almost as much expenditure as a hospice would. Perhaps more reproducible is the Symptom Control Team established at St Thomas's Hospital in London. This team is called in to advise on problems of pain or other distress by all the departments of the hospital. Needless to say, they have to be adept diplomats.

*

I hope I have made it evident that there is often room for improvement in the care of the dying in hospitals. With Dame Albertine Winner,[423] I can only chorus:

When all is said and done, it is good doctoring and good nursing that is needed more than anything else, so why don't we give it?

7. Dying Children

Only two in a hundred babies die in the first year of life. Most of these deaths will be in the first few hours as a result of congenital disease or obstetrical difficulties. Thereafter, nine out of ten of them will live past their fiftieth birthday. In all, some 27,000 children die in Britain each year. For centuries the death of children was part of family life, but is now a rarity in the richer countries. Dr Simon Yudkin, until recently a London paediatrician, reported only 95 deaths among 4,000 admissions to his wards. Of these children only nineteen were more than one year old, only eight experiencing a long and frightening illness.[434]

My own experience is limited to less than a dozen children who died in the hospices where I worked, so I shall have to draw heavily on the writings of others. Even then I have little to draw on, since very few doctors have enough experience to write about the death of children. Surgeons who specialize in correcting congenital deformities, and physicians concerned with treating leukaemia, are the only people who see many children die, and they never get used to it.

Even people who are accustomed to dealing with children, therefore, can be thrown off balance when a child is dying. Dr Yudkin wrote:

The dying child's questions and oblique references may not come to the parents or the consultant but to the registrar, houseman, schoolteacher, nurse, laboratory technician, or ward orderly. Should we all have reached a decision before the question is likely to be asked? Should we at least all have discussed it?

In this branch of terminal care more than in any other, a prior discussion among all concerned is needed.

A Child's Approach to Death

Children grieve over the loss of someone close to them in the way that adults do.* They seldom give a thought to their own death, however, unless they are worried by a morbid fear. Before the age of about three they have no concept of death at all. Thereafter their understanding depends on the attitude of those around them. If it is pretended that Grandad never died but 'went away' and when the subject is mentioned it is seen to embarrass the parents, then not only will a child pick up – for life – our modern taboo on death, but he may also imagine all kinds of terrifying things about it. These fantasies can be diverse and lurid. If they upset the child, he will need to be listened to carefully and gently, however much time it may take. This matter of time is vital because the child may only allude to his fears indirectly, and reassurance will have to be gentle and persistent. Doris Howell notes how much confidence can come from the use of well-tried liturgical prayers and services in the ward and sickroom.[168]

Maria Nagy asked nearly 400 children in Budapest what they thought death was.[261] She found that their replies indicated three stages of understanding:

The first is characteristic of children between three and five. They deny death as a regular and final process. Death is a departure, a further existence in changed circumstances. There are ideas too that death is temporary. Indeed distinction is made of degrees of death† ... Living and lifeless are not yet distinguished ...

In the second stage, in general between the ages of five and

---

* See p. 182.
† A man may be 'badly killed'.

nine,[355] death is personified, considered a person. Death exists but the children still try to keep it distant from themselves. Only those die whom the death-man carries off. Death is an eventuality. There also occur fantasies, though less frequently, where death and the dead are considered the same. In these cases they consistently employ the word death for the dead. Here death is still outside us and not universal ...

Finally, in the third stage, in general around nine years, it is recognized that death is a process which takes place in us, the perceptible result of which is the dissolution of bodily life. By then they know that death is inevitable. At this age not only the conception as to death is realistic, but also their general view of the world.

It is interesting to reflect whether these three stages represent increasing or decreasing understanding.

Attending a morbid funeral may spark off fears of death in a child, but most of them will talk freely and easily about the subject. Alison Player made the following observations:

A child may react variously and very strongly to the death of a member of his family, particularly the parent. Unconsciously he may feel the loss of his mother as a desertion, perhaps as a punishment for his own misbehaviour ... He may even feel that it is his own unconscious aggression to his parent which has killed him ... At the time of death very particularly, the child should have the opportunity to hear explanations of the truth given simply and calmly, his questions answered, and his feelings explicitly understood. The child is so vulnerable.[300]

Most children nowadays will never meet death, so it is usually a rather theoretical matter.[446] When facing their own premature death, however, it is nearly always found that it looks less of a threat to the child than does the separation from his parents involved in moving into hospital. Distress over anticipating painful medical procedures, or over the death of another child in the ward, have been found far to outweigh the fear of death in most children.[263] Research by Gerald Koocher[446] showed that 'there should be no unspoken barriers to this topic of conversation. Children are capable of talking about death, and seem to want to do this. They are pleased by the attention of understanding adults. Silence teaches them only that the topic is taboo; it cannot help them to cope with their feelings of loss.'

Dr Walter Alvarez tells how a slightly older age group – the teenagers – may react with great disappointment and bitterness to being told a grave prognosis;[9] but as he and another great American physician, Dr Alfred Worcester,* have pointed out, younger children die very easily.

The Approach of the Caring Team

Though labelled 'dying', they must remain as ordinary children, full of fun and wonder, not objects of pity or victims of cold scientific endeavour. Dr Cicely Saunders says:

I am sure I do not have to emphasize the importance of delight, of beauty and fantasy and of parties. This is the setting in which the patient can be allowed to talk, grumble or cry. This is the time when you talk about progress, about symptoms and their treatment, and allow questions. Fear is drained out of so many questions if they can be voiced.[333]

To enter a child's world and anticipate his fears and puncture the threat that seems to lodge in death, we have to be the very best people we know how to be. The following description of how the wise physician Sir William Osler behaved in the situation was recorded for us by another great doctor, Harvey Cushing:[75]

He visited our little Janet twice every day from the middle of October until her death a month later, and these visits she looked forward to with pathetic eagerness and joy ... Instantly the sickroom was turned into fairyland, and in fairy language he would talk about the flowers, the birds, and the dolls ... In the course of this he would manage to find out all he wanted to know about the little patient.

*See Bibliography.

The most exquisite moment came one cold, raw November morning, when the end was near, and he brought out from his pocket a beautiful red rose, carefully wrapped in paper, and told how he had watched this last rose of summer growing in his garden and how the rose had called out to him as he passed by that she wished to go along with him to see his 'little lassie'. That evening we had a fairy tea party, at a tiny table by the bed, Sir William talking to the rose, his little lassie and her mother in a most exquisite way ... and the little girl understood that neither fairies nor people could always have the colour of a red rose in their cheeks, or stay as long as they wanted to in one place, but that they nevertheless would be happy in another home and must not let the people they left behind, particularly their parents, feel badly about it; and the little girl understood and was not unhappy.

The secret is to give the child a sense of security, which means sharing with and trusting in someone else. 'A child separated from its mother may be quite safe – but it feels very insecure. A child in its mother's arms during an air-raid may be very unsafe indeed – but it feels secure.'[333]

If this trust is to grow, we must be strictly honest with children. They are much more alert than adults and detect lies easily.[18] Honesty means allowing the child to ask you, or tell you, anything he wishes. If bad news is to be given, this should be done with precision and tenderness. Idle or hasty reassurance cannot be precise, and is never tender. Neither, of course, is blurting out the 'whole truth'. If the child can trust those caring for him, and has the feeling that they are with him, on his side as it were, he will feel secure. If people try to avoid him or deceive him, he will feel vulnerable.[167] One way of helping the child to come to grips with his deterioration is to tell him exactly *how* it is happening, in as much scientific detail as he can comprehend. If he can then partake more intelligently in any further treatment that may be tried, he will feel less threatened. He should be allowed to exercise as much control as is practicable – dictating for instance who shall give his injections, regulating his own diet, taking his own medicines.[122]

To be able to face death with a child, we must first be honest with ourselves. Are we trying to reassure ourselves when we lie to him, or when we go on plying him with uncomfortable treatments even after the battle is clearly lost? Dr Yudkin pleads that we let the dying child die in peace. He says:

I am not, of course, referring to an acute crisis in illnesses which can perhaps be cured but, when the end is inevitable, although we feel the death of the child to be out of time, must we rush around with tubes, injections, masks and respirators? Someone said recently that no one nowadays is allowed to die without being cured. Perhaps we do it only for the parents' sake; but perhaps we ourselves cannot accept our limitations. And can we sometimes consider whether the dying child should be allowed to die at home?[434]

A lady whose son was born with major congenital abnormalities and lived for only one month, in a hospital, wrote to me as follows:

I am devoted to the paediatrician who looked after him and to the Sister who was in charge, and yet I think they handled his life and death wrongly. I was not with him when he died. I expressed milk for him but after a while was not allowed to breast feed him as I wished to. Photographs were taken of him, tubes inserted, his head shaved, etc. He did not die in peace and I feel in retrospect that I should have lived his life with him and been with him when he died. It is complicated, I know, because there must be cases when babies' lives are saved by giving them apparently inhumane treatment. Also, though my paediatrician took me into the ward at first, he thought it better for my husband and two elder children if I went home to them. But I always remember my mother's account of her own mother nursing a dying baby (in 1884 or thereabouts), sitting all night by the fire with the baby in her arms, and him dying like that. She never forgot, because she told her daughter about it so vividly, years later; and it seemed to me that if one's children must die, that is the way for it to happen.

The temptation to over-treat and over-protect is even

worse with children than with adults. There can be something of the atmosphere of a crusade, which is no more justified with children than with anyone else if it only procures them a worse death. Attention to the quality of a child's life is as vital as merely giving him more time. More time can be pointless if suffering fills it.

[Parents may feel too guilty to say that] they are saddened by the suffering to which we are contributing by persisting with cytotoxic drugs, platelet and blood transfusions and intravenous antibiotics, so that the child simply lives a life of transfusions. It requires sensitivity and absolute firmness, once the decision has been made at the highest team level that the condition is irrevocably out of control, to stick to it. The trouble is that clinicians can be ambivalent and so the parents don't say 'stop'. I've seen the whole family suffer while the terminal stage is prolonged.

By postponing natural death at this stage we only add to their suffering. Intravenous lines and naso-gastric tubes are irrelevant but too often are continued instead of concentrating on the relief of pain and the importance of play. – Dr Jennifer Chapman.[110]

Good terminal care has its place in paediatrics. The rules are the same. Pain (e.g. the awful bone pain in leukaemia) should be taken seriously and treated with four-hourly analgesics. Constipation is a serious risk; addiction is no risk at all. If the child is vomiting there is still no need to give injections: we have found an excellent analgesic for children is a half to one oxycodone suppository eight-hourly, usually with a paediatric 5 mg Stemetil suppository at the same time. At all times, the purpose for these medications should be explained to the child. (I find it helps to explain it to the mother first, so that she does not react defensively in front of the child and put him off.)

This approach does not preclude our being always on the lookout for signs of unexpected recovery. A cautionary tale from my own experience illustrates this. One of the London teaching hospitals sent a boy of eight to die in St

Joseph's Hospice. He had a growing brain tumour and had lapsed into unconsciousness. The only signs of life were sighing, breathing and an occasional moan. In the next bed was a retired taxi driver who died a few weeks later, and he 'adopted' the boy in a grandfatherly fashion. Passing the boy's bed one day, he remarked, 'I'm sure Hubert's asking for something.'

'Not when he's unconscious!' said the ward sister.

'Yes he is,' insisted Grandad, 'listen.' There followed a moan from Hubert.

'There you are!' came the triumphant exclamation. 'He wants some orange juice.'

Doubtfully Sister gave some in a feeding cup, and to everyone's surprise Hubert swallowed it and distinctly asked for more. So we pulled out his feeding tube and fed him by mouth. Gradually consciousness returned, limbs moved which had hitherto been flaccid. Energetic physiotherapy was instituted. Soon Hubert was taking walks in the garden with the staff nurse and having speech therapy. Once he could run he became the life and soul of the ward: imagine having twenty-two indulgent Grandads! The tea boy and general giver of cheek started taking weekends at home, then went to a school for delicate children, and finally back to completely normal living. He is in excellent health to this day.

The Parents

The first hint that all is not well will come to the child from a change in his parents' behaviour. He will find that he can get away with more naughtiness than usual, and that they do not let him out of their sight. They start to grieve and cannot hide it.[17]

Those caring for the family may have a very trying time. The parents often feel angry and want to blame someone bitterly: the family doctor did not diagnose what was wrong soon enough, the surgeon did not do the operation properly, the nurses did not make him comfortable enough, if Aunty Mary had not let them go swimming in the sea it would never have happened, if that car driver had kept to the speed limit ... and so on. All this will have to be patiently listened to like weathering a storm, because the repetition of the fears and frustrations to a listener enables them to develop insight. And this is how the process of healing begins for them.[147] Families who direct their frustration at the medical profession may turn to a clergyman for support. Those who feel angry with God will normally reject priests and look to the doctor. Both have to admit that they don't know all the answers.

Some families try to follow up every possibility of treatment. Certainly a visit to Lourdes, even if not followed by miracles, may be therapeutic for the whole family; but one should be wary of any expensive attempts at treatment which may cause distress to the young patient. There is no shortage of charlatans whose hocus pocus could be tried; some are sincere and some are positively mercenary.

The shorter the child's last illness, the sharper will be the reaction of the parents. Acceptance of the situation will be much easier for them if they have had time to grieve and adjust their outlook while he is still alive. This can be exasperating for the staff. Several times I had to calm the indignation of the nurses when the mother of a dying boy called Michael made complaints, or remade his bed, or hovered around interfering with nursing procedures. I had to impress on them the utter horror of the situation for her, and that she also was now our patient. In order that this grieving may be given time, and not come all in a flood, it is desirable that the parents are told of an inevitably fatal outcome at the earliest possible moment. But the first time they will probably take in very little of what is told them. It may all have to be repeated, without irritation, several times. To write it down for them may help.

To relieve his parents' frustration at feeling so impotent in the face of Michael's disease, we involved them as much as possible in his day-to-day care. Parents are very much part of the team. Not only should they be encouraged to help with the nursing, they may also want to be involved in the making of decisions. Some may prefer to leave all decisions to the doctor, particularly if they have a burden of guilty feelings to unload.[135] In one American hospital, 'Parents had regular educational conferences with the physicians in order to learn more about their children's diseases, the program of treatment, and the investigative program. The reception given by the parents was rewarding to the physicians.'[263] Every family will want to partake in the supervision of their child to a different degree. There will be a different balance point for each. For some almost anything other than passive visiting will be too painful. Others will feel as if they are deserting their duty if they do not contribute to every decision. How we found this balance point with one particular couple may perhaps be instructive.

Ann was unconscious, following a crash in a friend's car, and her condition was deteriorating. When admitted for terminal care she was found to have a chest infection. She did respond a little to stimulation, with a strange nasal cry. So one had to assume that some impressions were still received, which meant that she just might still be suffering. Of course she would be given full nursing care, but the question arose as to whether she should be given antibiotics for the potentially fatal chest infection. From the patient's point of view, it would probably have been kinder to relieve distress and allow the pneumonia to kill her gently. But we feared that the parents would feel guilty at having consented to her admission to the hospice if Ann died immediately. On the other hand they might be longing to see an end to her suffering. So we decided to hold a case conference.

The parents, the doctors and the ward sister accordingly met over a cup of tea. We explained to them that the neurosurgeon had found irreparable damage, but that we could probably keep Ann alive for years if we dosed her with drugs. At first they urged that everything possible be done, until her father realized that this was for their sake only, and not for hers. 'Will she always be like this?' he asked. This we confirmed and added that to preserve her life artificially *in this condition* for any length of time would feel wrong to us. The parents were certain that they wanted her present infection treated, just in case she showed any signs of recovery: they had not quite given up hope. Nevertheless, they also agreed that it would not be right to keep this going for years, and accepted that eventually we would have to stop treating her. 'But if you do decide not to treat her,' they said, 'just do what you think best without telling us, so that we don't have to think about it.' This perfect balance gave us a clear guide for the future and established firm trust between us all.

The end of the story is also salutary, because Ann showed some signs of improvement. Not only did she start to swallow again, but showed a distinct preference for being fed by her mother. Our hopes had risen so much that when she did develop another chest infection we had the dilemma all over again. In view of the improvement, we treated this infection as well. But this time the drugs failed to work: she had a series of fits and died. *L'homme propose, mais Dieu dispose.*

In his book *Death Comes Home*, the Rev. Simon Stephens lists four circumstances which can deepen the despair of the parents' grief: if the child were an only child, if surviving brothers or sisters showed disturbed behaviour due either to their own grief or to their receiving inadequate attention from distressed parents, if the death exacerbated some marital disharmony, or if the parents felt very guilty in connection with the child's death. As the Rev. Stephens says: *

The element of guilt is a common factor in parental grief. The failure to see a child across a busy main road, to check the brakes on a recently renovated pedal cycle, or to change well-

*p. 84: see Bibliography.

worn car tyres are just as likely to produce a guilt complex because of their disastrous consequences as is the suicide of a teenager. In such circumstances as these the element of guilt is always destructive and unless resolved in the company of a sympathetic friend may have grave repercussions.

The Society of Compassionate Friends* which the Rev. Stephens founded in Coventry now has branches all over Britain, enabling bereaved parents to meet and help one another. Its work has proved immensely valuable.

The tendency to idealize the dead is harmless provided that it does not encroach on our love for the living. 'In cases where the dead child has been "canonized" by his sorrowing parents to the exclusion of the other children,' the Rev. Stephens tells us, 'it has been shown that the siblings become antisocial in a desperate bid to attract attention and to win back their parents' love.' The mother may even have feelings of resentment towards her surviving children when they clamour for her notice, for she may feel that she owes it to the dead one to dwell morbidly on his loss. Alternatively she may become over-protective, fearing that a similar fate may overtake his brothers and sisters, and deny them half the adventures of childhood.

Home Care of the Dying Child

To have a seriously ill child at home can be reassuring for the child, but terrifying for the parents. It is essential that they have someone always available to call on for help. Many GPs will give a family their private number under these circumstances. Some hospitals employ a special liaison health visitor or paediatrician to visit the children at home, most promise immediate readmission if the family panic. Such emergencies as severe pain, vomiting or bleeding just cannot wait. Nothing reassures like competence. If the services laid on take hours to arrive, or if the GP uses the emergency call system out of

*Address on p. 186.

hours, home care may be impracticable. Much also depends on the maturity of the parents and whether they have a telephone.

Since many of the children live a long way from the treating hospital, there is obviously an urgent need for specialist care services in each community. A home care team for this purpose has been launched in London, Ontario,[84] and had we funds we would like to do the same in London, England. The number of children needing this care is increasing every year as treatment becomes possible for more of them.

At least home care enables parents to see they are essential to the child's care and not just pushed aside as helpless bystanders. This, and the deeper relationship possible, eases their grief afterwards. They need to be told not to neglect their other children, but to try to involve them also in the treatment routines. The parents will be more irritable than usual. If they have some insight into this, they will be able to apologize to the other children in the family and get them to understand. Very young children usually react by seeking attention with naughtiness. This has to be expected and to some extent tolerated. The patient's grandparents may also be difficult, with their theories as to why the illness occurred, their doubts about diagnoses and their fixed ideas about treatment. In particular they, as well as the parents, may be inclined to restrict the child's activity too much. What is actually needed from grandparents at this time is praise and encouragement for everyone in the situation.

Lindy Burton, in her excellent book,* explains that it is acceptability to their friends which concerns ill children. Their appearance and dress, therefore, needs attention. Schoolfriends should be encouraged to visit, and school studies continued as normally as possible.

Support in the community from GP, health visitor and district nurse can be made to look very amateur if the specialist team at the hospital do not keep them well in-

* See Bibliography.

formed. The ward sister should send a note home with the child, for the district nurse, inviting her to telephone. The GP will need to speak to the registrar or consultant, and to come back to them with any new problems that arise: a letter from them is insufficient. The hospital social worker could profitably liaise with the health visitor, who may be the only person likely to follow up the family after their child has died. Voluntary help in any neighbourhood is often best coordinated by the local clergyman, who may also have a role in supporting the father of the dying child. The fathers may value a man-to-man chat, and are often out at work in the hours that community nurses and social workers can visit.

Born Dying

When our baby daughter arrived and I took her from the midwife to hand to my wife, I just had to have a quick look for missing limbs, cleft lip, bifid spine and the like, in spite of myself. So much has been said recently about congenital deformities that many women have extreme anxiety until they have seen their new baby, and even so much as a contact with German measles sends them to their doctor in search of an abortion.

The vast majority of babies born with malformations live with them with only minor adjustments. But a few are incapable of independent existence, and soon die. In these cases the parents usually suffer a rather different kind of short, sharp grief.

Nowadays a few of these children pose a bizarre and torturing problem. Should they be resuscitated?[342] Should they be fed? Should their deformity be corrected by surgery in spite of probable mental deficiency? About 8% of all survivors of such operations are found to be severely handicapped and mentally affected. I am not in a position to decide on these questions: I can only repeat the arguments from opposing points of view.

Mr Ellison-Nash, a surgeon who operates on deformed

neonates and then maintains a profoundly loving follow-up at Chailey Heritage, avers that a surgeon with this skill should examine all cases, and operate whenever it is possible. He reasons that, when they are not operated on, these children do not all die, and it is not always possible to predict which ones will not. If they survive, their disabilities will be much worse than they would have been had operations been performed. For instance, children with hydrocephalus (a head swollen with fluid because the normal drainage channels are blocked) may go blind if an artificial valve is not inserted. They may then not die as expected.[104] He considers that the decision not to treat should only be taken when complications develop at the age of two or three in an infant who is showing signs of severe retardation.

Another surgeon, Mr Lloyd-Roberts, wrote:

We are confronted by a serious ethical problem in which the quantity of survival sometimes obscures the quality. The burden on the health and social services is immense.

The tragedy is emphasized when we compare the infant, the child and the young adult with severe paralysis. The infant differs little from his normal fellow—both are wet and must be carried everywhere. Even the child of six has some appeal, gallantly coping with his handicap with calipers, crutches and urinary bag. At thirteen he has usually reverted to a wheelchair in which he sits, obese, odiferous, acneiform and impotent, contemplating a sorry future with justifiable melancholy ... neglect, which includes the withholding of antibiotics, will usually resolve the dilemma.[221]

Officials of the Association for Spina Bifida* frowned on this pronouncement,[76] in particular the chairman for the Midlands, who said:

We should seriously consider the question of whether we are trying to produce a race of perfect human beings or taking the proper care of those we have ... As each supposedly hopeless

---

* Association for Spina Bifida and Hydrocephalus, Tavistock House North, Tavistock Square, London WC1 (01-388 1382).

case is treated, a little more is added to our knowledge of spina bifida, and to the chances of future generations of spina bifida children ... They should not be condemned because they pose a problem ...[426]

Usually the parents will partake in the decision[46] whether or not to treat. The dilemma of these parents was expressed by one mother as follows:

Few parents of spina bifida children are able to adopt the clear-cut views of some of your correspondents. We are more likely to be living in a perpetual cloud of conflicting feelings.

When my two-year-old son was born the team of doctors in charge thought his outlook was good and so operated immediately (they told me that if they did not operate he might not die but survive in a worse state). A year later we knew he would not only never walk but never even sit unsupported. Meanwhile he received from physiotherapists, doctors, social workers and all his family an immense amount of loving care. I think we all carry a double wish: that he will grow and prove intelligent and able to cope with life; and at the same time that he might die painlessly should life prove intolerable.

The emotional pendulum swings one way when we read of families who cope or of children who seem happy; and when we realize how much support and encouragement our society offers. It swings the other way when we read of the horrors of life for institutionalized adolescents, and realize how many people would like the problem swept away drastically. One day I think I am a moral coward for not being prepared to solve it by drastic means myself;[103] the next I reproach myself for insufficient courage and optimism in thinking of the future.

There is certainly a good case for leaving spina bifida children unoperated at birth (though I wonder how many doctors would leave their own children); but I suspect that some of those who advance it are trying to tidy up the world in a way that can never be done. What about mongol children, spastics, children injured in accidents? In hospital waiting rooms I have been *envied* by other mothers for my bright strong-armed little boy ...

The whole controversy may be resolved in the next few years by improvement in the accuracy of prediction of a deformed child's chances of survival and health, but it is more likely that the criteria determining treatment will continue to depend on the philosophy of the individual surgeon.[209] Sitting in judgement over such criteria is easy for those not obliged to take these awful decisions, and frankly I think such self-appointed moralizers should be quiet.

Open Questions

I can only echo Dr Simon Yudkin in saying that in our care of dying children we still find more questions than answers. Because we are at a loss as to how relief can be brought to the child, we often concentrate on the parents instead – and certainly we have much help to offer them. But a genius to equal Osler and his wonderful approach is sadly wanting – we await wisdom. What will certainly not do is the coldly scientific attitude which thinks that pat answers to human problems can be found by analyses of data alone, however essential these may be to verify the insights of wisdom. Many papers reveal this shallow approach, using such sick expressions as 'a human love object' and 'family homeostasis' as a substitute for accurate observation. When we approach dying children we must do so with deep humility and open hearts, however much it hurts.

8. The Right Time to Die

So when at last the Angel of the darker drink
Of Darkness finds you by the river-brink,
And, proferring his Cup, invites your Soul
Forth to your lips to quaff it – do not shrink.

Rubaiyat of Omar Khayyam

The duty of a doctor is to restore his patients to health. For some he cannot do this, but he can keep them at least in reasonable shape, jogging along as functioning individuals. But for some others he can do neither: for these the *healthy* thing to do is to die.

It is proposed that there is a right time to die; that this time may come before a man has breathed the very last breath of which his body is capable; and that an experienced physician can recognize, or learn to recognize, that this right time to die has come. Please understand that what is proposed is to refrain from prolonging life beyond the right time, NOT to hasten the termination of life in any way. I will deal with euthanasia in the next chapter. What worries people, particularly nurses, is the prospect of the senile and suffering being kept alive, and not the question of euthanasia at all: that is just a red herring.[268]

This is a problem without precedent, since we have acquired the ability significantly to delay death only in this century. There are no traditional ethics in medicine, in the church, or in the law, to guide us in problems related to resuscitation and terminal care.

Watching a patient and responding appropriately to his

real needs is so much more intelligent and precise than a blunderbuss type of medicine which mechanically applies a standard treatment for each diagnosis, irrespective of the patient's age, health or maturity. Lord Amulree coined the term 'medicated survival', and made a plea for medical students to be taught what are the limits of treatment.[10] They must be shown that a man's death does not represent a humiliating defeat of medicine, but is the logical conclusion to life.[94] To die well is a great achievement, a very positive step which makes a man so much the greater, so much more completely a man. Good terminal care will enable him to take this step – that is what it is all about.[336]

Elderly people will often make the point that they are quite ready to die, and find the prospect not in the least alarming.[299] A change of mind which is not resignation, but preparation, becomes evident as death approaches. Active treatment and attempts at vigorous mobilization would now be out of place. Just because we can do something at this stage, it does not follow that it is either right or kind always to do it.[329] When a patient is seen to be preparing for death, this is something we should respect. It is not at all the same thing as the wilful decision of the suicide, or the arrogant demand of the euthanasiast, but a real change in the man's outlook and understanding. A trust, a relaxation, a contentment, a willing giving up, are all evident. If a patient who is dying does not take this step, which is the last big step of life, then one should seriously consider whether one's care was deficient. It is a legitimate medical decision to abandon *cure*, but never to abandon *care*.

I remember how, when my grandmother realized that she had a breast cancer (in 1960, before the present higher rate of cure for this condition), she drew out her savings from the bank and went on an expensive shopping spree. My mother was puzzled, but accompanied her as she bought shoes, silk stockings, lacy underwear, a smart costume, matching hat and handbag and a pair of white gloves. They were all carefully stored in drawers and cupboards (with mothballs, I'm afraid!), and the mystery deepened. Then, on the day of her death, she asked to be fully decked out in the whole outfit 'because I'm going before God today'. She was too busy with these preparations to be worried about the actual process of dying.

A Mrs P. whom I knew had evaded difficulties throughout her life. With much help from the hospice team, however, she faced them all in her last three months of life. There was a problem with her two daughters: the elder had been her favourite, so that her relations with the younger one were cold and strained. With psychiatric help she was able to open up to the girl for the first time, and be friends. Mrs P. cross-examined me about her cancer several times, always indicating what reply she wanted. But the last time, she put up no defences at all, and just asked 'Am I dying?' She insisted that I should be honest, and she showed great interest, but was in no way upset. Later that week she saw the chaplain, at my suggestion, because she had made some comment about Judgement which I thought was more in his province. Having thus come slowly to terms with the family, her disease, and finally with God, she died at the right time of pneumonia, which we did not try to cure.

The Old Man's Friend

I would wish that the young doctor have deeply impressed on his mind the real limits of his art, and that when the state of his patient gets beyond this, his office is to be a watchful but quiet spectator of the operations of nature. – Thomas Jefferson

When not to treat is usually self-evident.[1] Apart from anything else, doctors are not as powerful as the layman often thinks. The decision to treat an elderly person's pneumonia is no guarantee of cure. It becomes obvious to any geriatrician that while some patients are treatable, others have lived their allotted span, and cannot be resurrected by any treatment. Geriatric decisions need to be based on common sense and compassion, rather than on a spirit of adventure.

Sir William Osler called bronchopneumonia 'The Old Man's Friend' because it is the usual ultimate cause of death for someone already weakened by a chronic disease (p. 84). The fear that we may banish this friend from the bedside is not well founded, since treatment often fails, but it is our efforts to banish him which can give patients great discomfort. Treatment with antibiotics is much more likely to be successful when the younger sufferer from advanced cancer contracts pneumonia. The results can be catastrophic, if doctors have their priorities wrong and tacitly accept longevity as the aim, at any price.[45] We certainly need good techniques, but as Sir Theodore Fox pointed out,[164] we also need to know when to use them.

In a case like this the first decision that has to be made is whether the illness is terminal. If it is regarded as such, the whole caring team then becomes involved in a combined effort to bring comfort to the patient as he dies. Decisions should now be taken collectively: the nurses, chaplain, physiotherapist and relatives should all be consulted. There can be no absolute rules with so fine a creature as a Man, and in some cases the decision will be the patient's own. For some people death will be a quick release, for others the dignified way to die will be in fighting to the last.

A doctor may have to be gently firm over his decision to refrain from meddlesome therapy, because nurses or relatives may press him to *do* something if, for instance, a dying patient's breathing becomes laboured. This may be uncomfortable to watch, but the patient is usually unconscious in the final stages of terminal pneumonia, and any treatment given at this stage would be therapy for the watchers rather than for the patient. To secure a peaceful end for the patient, the doctor or ward sister may have to point out that interference at this point would be what

Sir George Pickering called 'false charity'. One doctor even dubbed penicillin – the mainstay of treatment for pneumonia – 'the old man's enemy!'[13]

When to Resuscitate?

> Is life a boon? If so it must befall
> That death, whene'er he call,
> Must call too soon.
>
> Is life a thorn? Then count it not a whit!
> Then count it not a whit –
> Man is well done with it.

W.S. Gilbert in *The Yeoman of the Guard*

Dying is normal – a healthy thing to do; everyone does it! Death is not an enemy to be swatted and parried to the last grim moment.

When I was a junior physician in a hospital, we were once called urgently to the bedside of a lady of ninety. The nurse used the term 'cardiac arrest' – the old lady's heart had stopped (as hearts are apt to do, around ninety!). But because the cardiac arrest alarm was raised, I and the other houseman launched into a full-scale resuscitation. With violent drugs injected direct into the heart, blasts of electric current through her chest, noise and chaos, she had anything but a peaceful death. On reflection we realized that all this had been inappropriate, but nothing in our medical student training gave us any guide. Indeed once the feeling of emergency is in the air, there is not time to weigh up the pros and cons. The decision is rarely a doctor's anyway, because usually the only person on the scene when an emergency occurs is a nurse – probably a relatively junior one if it is night-time – and she decides whether or not to resuscitate. Needless to say, it is a courageous nurse who decides not to. Once things have started, it is very difficult for the doctor when he arrives to stop everything, particularly if the patient is showing signs of reviving.

Clearly, what is required is a prior discussion, involving the whole team, to consider just to what *kind* of life they would be restoring the patient. They must ask themselves, 'Are we hoping to return the patient to health, or are we to regard his illness as terminal so that, if he dies, he is to be left in peace and not resurrected?'[293] For the patient with a less dramatic form of fatal illness – say a spreading cancer or a progressive paralysis like motor neurone disease – a similar question needs to be answered: 'What is our aim with this particular patient?'

If no definite answer presents itself, then one will institute what Professor Duncan Vere called a 'trial of therapy'.[388] Treatment of the patient's condition is started, and he is watched closely to see if it helps. If no progress is made, then the treatment is discontinued at once. The parallel is in midwifery, where the obstetrician watching beside someone who, he anticipates, may have difficulty in childbirth, allows a 'trial of labour'. At the first sign of anything going wrong he abandons the trial for a Caesarian operation.

It is easy to hope for omnipotence from doctors, but when all is said and done it is good nursing which keeps people alive more than any medical pyrotechnics. Many a pneumonia is fatal in spite of antibiotics, and many resolve in spite of not being treated. Even the most bizarre and violent treatments give very limited returns in terms of lengthened life. One American paper tells a series of stories of patients with terminal illnesses who were rehabilitated (aged 92, with a fractured hip, pneumonia and senile dementia), force fed (aged 86, with a collapsed spine and too weak to fight off the feeding nurses), and resuscitated (aged 80, with a stroke which left him mute and paralysed, followed by a second one which rendered him comatose). Here are two passages from the third of these case histories:

The attending physician was ensnared in the family's death wishes and provided a vacuum of medical and nursing guidance. Indeed, he expressed his desire to the nursing staff that nothing be done for the patient: 'The patient is terminal and should be permitted to die peacefully.'

The nursing staff, however, had become attached to the patient during his stay at the institution. They insisted they be permitted to feed the patient and engage in a total nursing care program, including restorative care.

The director of nursing received permission from the medical director of the institution to address her wishes to the attending physician on the basis that the *nursing staff had a clear commitment to maintain life* [my italics] and was under no obligation to be the agent of the death wishes of family or physician. The attending physician relented and permitted the nursing staff to feed the patient via nasogastric tube, thus providing an adequate intake of fluid and electrolytes, calories, vitamins and medication. A restorative nursing program, including physical therapy, was instituted ... The patient was once again able to be transferred from bed to chair and to ambulate with assistance in the parallel bars. He expired five months later from an additional massive stroke.[250]

This idea that doctors and nurses must preserve life at all costs is an odd one, and quite new. Never has this been their duty. The famous Hippocratic Oath required a doctor to swear by the God of Health, but not by Life. His concern should always be with the good health of the whole man, not with the longevity of his body.[265]

The principle to guide us in decisions about life and death was (and I write as a non-Catholic) beautifully delineated by Pope Pius XII,[298] who distinguished between ordinary and extraordinary measures. Ordinary treatment means whatever a patient can obtain and undergo without thereby imposing an excessive burden on himself or others.[27]

It is only experience which can teach a doctor how to discriminate in this kind of situation. Not long ago we thought that a flat electro-encephalogram (i.e. the absence of any electrical activity in the brain) indicated that a man was dead. Now every intensive care unit has stories of people who were comatose with a flat E.E.G., and apparently dead for weeks or even months, and then began to recover. The question of when to turn off the intravenous drips and respirators whereby the patient with brain damage is artificially given food and breath has thus been hit back into the doctor's court. No rules are available. He can only say that if there is no brain activity for some time (how long depending on the extent of physical damage to the patient), and the patient's condition looks as if it is deteriorating, the time has come to turn off.[149] It is obvious that the machines have to be stopped at some point, otherwise beds would be used for years in maintaining corpses while waiting lists of the living grew longer.[204] The medical dilemma was made public in the world-famous case of Karen Quinlan, who lapsed into irreversible coma in April 1975.[97] This resulted in an endless debate with many published opinions about it[134] and, in America, where doctors enjoy much less trust from patients than we do in Britain, a rash of protective legislation.[245] This ranges from clandestine efforts to legalize euthanasia to attempts to clarify the legal position of a doctor whose patient refuses further treatment. The Natural Death Act in California was the first, and has made little impact on actual medical practice in spite of stirring up a considerable debate.[188]

Willy-nilly we are being forced by events to face up to situations in which our only guide is clinical judgement. As an editorial in the *Lancet* said,

> It is part of the clinician's duty to recognize the inevitability of death in certain situations and to avoid the unnecessary physical and emotional trauma associated with unsuccessful attempts at resuscitation ...[206]

The same applies to surgeons, who have been admonished not to operate on the elderly without very good cause. Sir David Smithers said,

> It is no great tribute to the art of surgery to see a feeble old gentleman dragging out his life for a few months cured of an

advanced pharyngeal carcinoma* if deprived of many things which might have made these few months tolerable.

His words were echoed by Sir Stanford Cade, another distinguished surgeon.[54] There is even a limit to what nurses should attempt. Forcibly to feed the dying robs them of dignity, and nurses are sometimes very worried by the forcible administration of drugs. Indeed, this has already led to the scandalous dismissal of one hospital sister who declined to give an antibiotic to an aged patient who refused it. The doctor argued that as the patient was confused, other people should decide what was good for her. But the sister said that the lady's decision was a very reasonable one. 'Why are you making me have these medicines, you cruel one?' she asked. Under the circumstances it was incumbent upon the doctor to inject the drugs forcibly himself – nurses should certainly never be obliged to do anything against their conscience. In a book produced by the Medical Protection Society,† J. Leahy Taylor even went as far as to say, 'It can hardly be thought proper to deprive a patient of the right to decline consent solely because he happens to be detained under the Mental Health Act.'

The Legal Position

Anyone who is worried that treatment to themselves or a relative may constitute 'meddlesome medicine' should discuss this with their own doctor. It may also help to contact the Patients' Association, which may be able to investigate the case.

In 1961 a case was considered in Sweden, where a Dr Sallin stopped the intravenous drip treatment of a lady in her eighties who had an irreversible cerebral haemorrhage.[180] Not until February 1965 was he finally acquitted of charges of killing.

No real test cases have yet come before British courts,

* Cancer of the upper throat. † *The Doctor and the Law*, 1970, p. 99.

but of course we are free to refuse any medical treatment at any time. It is supposed that if a doctor was sued for assault by a patient whom he had revived when that patient had refused treatment and hoped to die, the court might uphold the doctor. He would, however, have to show that there was an element of confusion in the patient's other behaviour at the time. If the patient was resuscitated against his will without being consulted, he would probably be awarded '$\frac{1}{2}$p damages'. In America, however, in some States it has been upheld that a doctor in these circumstances is guilty of assault, while in other States patients or relatives appealing to a judge when doctors refused to discontinue life-support therapy have been waved aside.[444] There is confusion.[211]

In English Common Law, all surgery or administration of potent drugs technically constitutes an assault whether the patient consents or not, so that any kind of medicine can only be justified by appeal to the 'Doctrine of Necessity'. This requires that the evil averted be greater than the evil performed. Obviously this applies to all routine surgery.[193] Also it is asserted that only as much evil may be done as is reasonably necessary to avert the greater evil. Thus a surgeon had to defend himself energetically in court when, in the course of removing a gall bladder, he incidentally removed the patient's appendix as well. (He was acquitted, but only because he could present statistics to show that an inflamed gall bladder frequently disturbs the health of the appendix as well.)

The withdrawal of useless treatment to avoid prolonging the process of dying could be justified by the doctrine of necessity,[254] and so could the giving of treatment which, in relieving the suffering of the dying, would possibly hasten their demise. Euthanasia could not be so justified, as we shall see in the next chapter.

This story, entitled 'Fools Rush In', appeared in the Christmas edition of the *Guy's Hospital Gazette* in 1969:

'Pertinax,' said Aunt Agatha. 'Are you now a Real Doctor?'
'Yes, aunt,' replied Pertinax, 'If this evening the cry went up,

"Is there a doctor in the house?" it would be my duty to respond.' Aunt Agatha muttered something that sounded like 'Fools rush in,' and applied herself to her programme.

Pertinax glanced idly round the concert hall; it was definitely not his idea of a celebration to see Sir Bultitude Baton conducting on his hundredth birthday, but Aunt A. was not a bad old trout and had sound views on food and drink; her choice of seats was less satisfactory, from the upper box it was impossible to see the face of the girl with the gorgeous hair in the second violins. However, he had had a good dinner, was pleasantly drowsy, and could contemplate his future glorious career in peace. (... 'Sir Pertinax Perforans was mercifully present on this occasion, and at the famous performer's side in a moment' ...) Sir Bultitude took his place amidst the plaudits of the audience; cellos led the orchestra into the dreamy strains of the first movement, Pertinax following them into the rosy glow of the future.

Suddenly, there was a crash and Pertinax started up to see that the tympani had, on this occasion, been augmented by the contact of Sir Bultitude's spare form with the platform. It was a matter of seconds only for Pertinax to leap from the box and, snatching a trumpet from its astonished owner, to sink on his knees by the side of the unconscious centenarian. Heart sounds came there none. Beckoning to the First Horn, as having a good respiratory excursion, he demonstrated in less than four seconds the most efficient method of administering the Kiss of Life, and started to open Sir Bultitude's shirt. This was, unfortunately, impossible to do at short notice, as the wearer was of the old school and the front was inseparable from the studs owing to its resemblance to sheet-iron. There was not a moment to be lost, so Pertinax merely tore off the tie and wing collar, and applied himself to cardiac massage through the glacial expanse, occasionally reminding the First Horn that it was unnecessary to turn this particular recipient of his breath over from time to time to 'empty him out'.

Minutes passed, the First Horn had been replaced by the Second, then by the Trumpets, followed by the Woodwinds, and Pertinax began to realize that even he might soon have to call upon the Kettledrum to relieve him for a short space. The rest of the orchestra sat mute, the audience silent and amazed, reporters were writing shorthand at a tremendous speed, and even a quiet little man who had come on the platform murmuring 'Sir Bultitude's personal geriatrician' was stunned into inaction by the brilliance of Pertinax's technique.

After what seemed like hours, Sir Bultitude stirred, his right hand straying feebly towards his chest. Signing to the Piccolo to desist, Pertinax bent down to catch the barely audible syllables from the trembling lips. 'Angels ... fear ...' Of course, thought Pertinax, the old man could not realize his deliverance, and was fumbling for some religious medal. Tenderly the young man slipped his hand beneath the now battered shirt-front and drew out a small disc, a gesture which brought forth tumultuous applause from the over-tensed audience and orchestra, and as he did so, his eyes fell upon the words 'Please do *not*, repeat *NOT* attempt resuscitation.' As the eyes of Sir Bultitude opened and fixed him with a venomous stare Pertinax closed his own.

The thunderous applause continued, and Pertinax felt a sharp poke in his ribs: 'Wake up,' said Aunt Agatha's voice. Pertinax opened his eyes and looked down on the platform where Sir Bultitude was shaking hands with the leading Violin. 'I think we will go down to the bar,' said Aunt Agatha; Pertinax agreed.

It was Thomas Jefferson, at the age of seventy-three, who wrote to a friend, 'I enjoy good health: I am happy in what is around me, yet I assure you I am ripe for leaving all, this year, this day, this hour.' This readiness for death is common in the elderly. I recall waking up old Mrs McP. after her first night in the hospice. She peeped over the bedclothes at me with wondering eyes, looking at my white coat, the white sheets and the white uniforms of the nursing nuns. With breathless delight she asked me, 'Am I in 'eaven?'

The Last Enemy

The last words of the great surgeon William Hunter, whispered to a friend as he lay dying, were, 'If I had strength to hold a pen I should write how easy and pleasant a thing it is to die.'

MED A 521153
5

BIRTHS AND DEATHS REGISTRATION ACT 1953
(Form prescribed by the Registration of Births Deaths, and Marriages Regulations 1968)

MEDICAL CERTIFICATE OF CAUSE OF DEATH

For use only by a Registered Medical Practitioner WHO HAS BEEN IN ATTENDANCE during the deceased's last illness, and to be delivered by him forthwith to the Registrar of Births and Deaths

	Registrar to enter No. of Death Entry

Name of deceased *Mrs. Mary* ×××××××

Date of death as signed to me *2nd* day of *April* 19*70* Age as stated to me *84*

Place of death *Raphael Ward, St. Joseph's Hospice, London E.8.*

Last seen alive by me *1st* day of *April* 19*70*

{1 The certified cause of death takes account of
   information obtained from post-mortem.
2 Information from post-mortem may be available later.*
3 Post-mortem not being held.

(a) Seen after death by me.
(b) Seen after death by another medical practitioner
   but not by me.
(c) Not seen after death by a
   medical practitioner.

	These particulars not to be entered in death register
CAUSE OF DEATH	Approximate interval between onset and death

I
Disease or condition directly leading to death† ···· ····   *(a) She died of old age*
                          due to (or as a consequence of)
Antecedent causes.
Morbid conditions, if any, giving   *(b)*
rise to the above cause stating the   *due to (or as a consequence of)*
underlying condition last.   *(c)*

II
Other significant conditions, contributing to the death, but not related
to the disease or condition causing it.   II

I hereby certify that I was in medical attendance during the above named deceased's last illness, and that the
particulars and cause of death above written are true to the best of my knowledge and belief.

Signature *R. Lamerton*   Qualifications as *MB.S.S. L.R.C.P*
                              registered by
                              Medical Council

Residence *St. Joseph's Hospice, E.8.*   Date *2.4.70*

* Please ring appropriate digit and letter.
† This does not mean the mode of dying, such as heart failure, asphyxia, asthenia, etc.: it means the disease, injury, or complication which caused death.

SEE BACK

MED A 521153
5

NOTICE TO INFORMANT

I hereby give notice that I have this day signed
a medical certificate of the cause of death
of *Mrs. Mary* ×××××××

Signature *R. Lamerton*

Date *2.4.70*

This notice must be given by the Certifying Medical
Practitioner to the person who is qualified and liable
to act as informant for the purpose of the registration
of the death. As to the person liable to act as
informant, see back.

DUTIES OF INFORMANT

This notice is to be delivered by the informant to the
registrar of births and deaths for the sub-district in
which the death occurred. The death cannot be registered until the medical certificate has reached the
registrar. Failure to deliver this notice to the registrar
renders the informant liable to prosecution.

*The informant must be prepared to state accurately
to the registrar the following particulars:—*

(1) The date and place of death, and the deceased's
usual address, (2) the full names and surname, (and
the maiden surname if the deceased was a woman who
had married), (3) the date and place of birth (town
and country; or country if born abroad), (4) the
occupation (and the name and occupation of her
husband if the deceased was a married woman or a
widow), (5) whether deceased was in receipt of a
pension or allowance from public funds and (6) if
deceased was married, (he age of the surviving widow
or widower.

**DECEASED'S MEDICAL CARD MUST
BE DELIVERED TO THE REGISTRAR**

Figure c

133

It is our modern evasion of the subject and utter refusal even to believe in it that is at the root of some of our crazy attempts to resurrect the very aged. All kinds of errors follow as we attempt to conceal death from ourselves, from society and from the dying themselves. Sedation with drugs at the approach of death, for instance, if instituted for the sole purpose of preventing the dying person from dying consciously, is a regrettable practice, particularly for religious patients.[118]

One particular denial which amused me arose when an old lady died after a long period in a geriatric home. She had no particular fatal illness, but had just faded out normally and peacefully, so on the death certificate I wrote 'She died of old age'. It is reproduced in this book (Figure C) because I still have it: the Registrar returned it to me, objecting that I had not written down an acceptable diagnosis. If I did not change it, the Coroner would carry out an autopsy examination and *find* a diagnosis. So I let the official concerned dictate a proposed diagnosis to me, and I put it in inverted commas. I would have liked to pursue this comic turn to its illogical conclusion, but a post mortem examination would have distressed the family. The incident underlines, however, to what extent our present-day society fears death: in the modern view it is pathological, not normal: it is horrible, not welcome: it is not allowed on the National Health!

The Captives (By 'E.R.T.', in the *Nursing Mirror*, 17.12. 71)

> 'Our scene is over; let us go home now.'
> 'No, no,' said they, 'for us it's not half done;
> We do not want the end, so why should you?'
> 'Because,' we said, 'we're ready to be gone.'
>
> 'Into the dark?' they cried, 'no, stay with us;
> Into that fearful dark you shall not go.
> Once you go there, you never will return;
> Last time you started out, we drew you back.'

We pleaded with them. 'Let us go this time;
Those we have loved are gone. We hear them now,
Waiting to fetch us through the dark to light.
Our time has come; we do not want to stay.'

'But stay you must and shall,' the answer came,
'For we can hear no voices calling you.
Beside, we would not have it said of us
"They let some geriatric patients die"!'

We were not asking for a lethal drug,
To go before our scene is fully played.
Just to make our exit on our proper cue,
Leaving the stage with grace and dignity.

But our custodians cannot understand.
Deaf to the voices, they still hold us back
From that sweet dark where friendly hands are stretched.
They are so clever; we, so old and tired.

9. The Euthanasia Debate

Since I cannot put the case for euthanasia with much conviction, I would refer the reader to the Bibliography at the back of this book for works which put the case cogently and forcefully.

As I understand it the humanist wants to control life and death. He wants to be kept alive until he decides to go, and then have euthanasia administered. This idea is based on a truth, hence its power. Men do have the freedom to make and execute this decision, because at their full stature, men are gods (Psalm 82 : 6 and John 10 : 30–38 confirm this for any Christian among my readers who may need such confirmation). It is, however, rare for a man to stand at his full stature, particularly when smitten by pain and disease. Some would choose to live too long – and as I pointed out in the previous chapter, there is a right time to die. Others would decide to die as a variation on running away. Now they emigrate to New Zealand; euthanasia, like suicide, would give them an even more distant haven.

Man is so much more natural than the humanist supposes. He does not have to conquer Nature, only to obey her, for his maximum happiness and freedom. We do not fly aeroplanes, for example, by conquering the air, but by obeying its laws of aerodynamics.

Definitions

The word 'euthanasia' comes from the Greek for a good death. Nowadays it does not mean that, but has a more precise connotation.[153] It involves one person killing another, either to relieve him of suffering which could not be relieved by any other means, or because he does not appear to be capable of sanity. Let us consider what euthanasia is and what it is not: [201]

1. In the days before morphine and similar opiate pain-killers were used properly, such large doses sometimes had to be given to relieve pain that the breathing was also suppressed. This side-effect often shortened the patient's life. The Pope[297] and other moralists,[273] the law and medical ethics, all considered this practice to be both moral and praiseworthy. This hastening of death was never an example of euthanasia, because the treatment was not designed to kill. If death did result, it was an unavoidable side-effect. The situation is nowadays of theoretical interest only, since it is medically inexcusable to use pain-killers so clumsily. As explained on pages 47 and 89, modern methods of pain control do not shorten life, and seldom even impair consciousness. It has often been suggested that doctors deliberately overdosed the patient with morphine, and that legalizing euthanasia would only be acknowledging what is already going on. But a doctor who wanted to kill someone could do it much more effectively and less obviously than that. Morphine would be a hopelessly blunt instrument for the job, and would have to be given in really enormous doses. This is not common medical practice, and never has been. In recent years two doctors attempted to kill patients with drugs which included morphine.[41] Both failed.

2. The withdrawing of artificial means of prolonging life was dealt with in the previous chapter. This is not euthanasia, it is just good medicine. It is already legal and no change in the law is required.[117] It is merely acting upon a recognition that a test – a trial of therapy – has yielded a negative result.

3. To refrain from giving inappropriate treatment is not euthanasia either. For instance, if a man has lost a large

slice of brain in a road accident, but still goes on breathing, he should not be given antibiotics to prevent infection of the wound! It is a legitimate medical judgement to decide that it is not in the interest of the patient to resuscitate him.

4. Suicide is another form of killing. This has not been a crime in Britain since 1961, because we cannot lay upon a man the duty always to be rational and never to be depressed. The duty (a moral, not a legal duty) lies with others to prevent him reaching a suicidal state. But if other people are not around when he does try to kill himself, so runs the reasoning, it would be cruel to brand him a criminal.

5. What *is* illegal is assisted suicide,[359] with carefully-defined exceptions in some countries. If one person urges or helps another to kill himself, this is a crime. The logic of the law's position is simple: a man strong enough to kill himself is strong enough to meet and survive adversity provided he is given enough help. If I find a man about to commit suicide, it is my duty to urge him not to do it, to care for him in such a way that he does not want to do it, and to put him in touch with social agencies that will ensure that he does not need to do it. If I just agree and help him, it is because I am too lazy to care and to fulfil my duty towards him. And afterwards, who could be sure I had not murdered him?[cf. 418]

6. Voluntary euthanasia is homicide by request, the person doing the killing being a doctor or nurse, and the person doing the requesting being the patient himself. The legalization of this measure was proposed in the House of Lords in 1936 by Lord Ponsonby,[142] using a bill largely drawn up by the President of the Society of Medical Officers of Health, Dr C. Killick Millard.[247] This gentleman founded the Euthanasia Society which in 1969 changed its name to the Voluntary Euthanasia Society, and is now called 'Exit'. The matter was discussed again in the Lords in 1950, when Lord Chorley moved for Papers,[143] but it was not until 1969 that another Bill was put before

the House, this time by Lord Raglan.[144] In 1970 Hugh
Gray, M.P. asked permission to bring in a Private Member's Bill to the House of Commons, but leave was not
granted.[141]

The debate was revived in the Lords in 1976 when Lady
Wootton suggested that assisted suicide be legalized.[173] In
a brilliant debate[145] the proposal was squashed by a bigger
majority than had voted against any previous euthanasia
Bill. Later in the same year the Criminal Law Revision
Committee considered the possibility of bringing into the
law a new class of homicide, called 'mercy killing'.[60] This
would apply to a person who, from compassion, unlaw-
fully killed another person who was, or was believed by
him to be, (1) permanently subject to great bodily pain
and suffering; or (2) permanently helpless from bodily or
mental incapacity; or (3) subject to rapid incurable bodily
or mental degeneration.[100] The Editor of the *Daily Telegraph*[77] commented on this idea as follows: '... the more
crucial objection is the age old argument against requiring juries to direct their minds to the assessment of motives
rather than intentions. Who is to say whether Aunt Jane
was consigned to her Maker for the sake of her health or
for her money, or even in deference to the sociological
theories of some homicidal philanthropist?'

Most of these attempts to alter the Law of England
were concerned only with voluntary euthanasia. This
would be administered to those suffering severely from
incurable disease. The patient concerned would have to
sign a form requesting euthanasia. If he still wanted it one
month later, a doctor could kill him, or if he ratified his
decision three years later, the declaration would remain
in force for the rest of his life unless he revoked it.

7. Involuntary euthanasia has also been suggested.[129]
Professor Glanville Williams defended the idea of its use
for 'hopelessly defective infants' (*Euthanasia and the
Right to Death*, ed. A. B. Downing, p. 145 – see Bibliography). Lord Ailwyn, speaking in support of Lord Raglan's Bill, said it mercifully lit a torch *in the right direc-*

tion (my italics). He had just visited a low standard geriatric ward, and described it with horror. 'Here it was,' he said, 'in all its pathetic reality, the crying need to offer these poor creatures the one remedy one felt in one's bones that they might accept gratefully and thankfully grasp.' He said it was a melancholy thought to 'withhold from them this boon, this milk of human kindness' – 'to be wafted painlessly into the life to come'. Quoting the words of St Paul, Lord Ailwyn suggested that euthanasia would be the ultimate charity: 'And now abideth faith, hope, charity, these three; but the greatest of these is charity.' Charity of this mighty order would effectively knock out the faith and hope! Lord Ailwyn's final solution would be such a saving to the nation, because we would never have to bother with good geriatric care (the other solution).[42]

Lord Chorley also, when initiating the debate in 1950, said, 'Another objection is that the Bill* does not go far enough, because it applies to adults and does not apply to children who come into the world blind, deaf and crippled, and who have a much better case than those for whom the Bill provides. That may be so, *but we must go step by step.*' (My italics.)

'In the course of time euthanasia would,' suggested Miss Mary Rose Barrington of the Voluntary Euthanasia Society executive, 'reach the same state as kidney transplants at the present time ... we may expect soon to pass from a "contracting in" to a "contracting out" position. A good death will not come to people in general until the climate of opinion shows clearly that people want to be helped out at the end, whether or not they can bring themselves to talk about it.'[25]

The argument that legalization of voluntary euthanasia would be the thin edge of a wedge is unquestionably valid: that is the expressed intention of its proponents. Suggestions such as these prompt many people, notably Roman Catholics, to say that voluntary euthanasia would just be softening the public resistance to much more

*i.e. the 1936 one.

dangerous legislation.[79] Clearly their fears are not groundless, particularly when you consider the escalation of abortion following the 1967 Act.[124]

8. To complete the list I will mention that killing someone in self defence or in war has always been accepted as legal, and death due to carelessness ranks as manslaughter, not murder. Capital punishment is still practised in some countries. It was discontinued in Britain not because it was inconvenient, a poor deterrent or used in error, but just because it was considered a barbarous solution to crime.[116] In the same way, I suggest that euthanasia would be a barbarous solution to suffering.

9. Finally, murder and genocide are universally accepted as wrong. It is interesting to reflect that it is not easy to say just why they are wrong – the best reason being simply because we all feel it is wrong. This natural inhibition is the basis of civilization, and deeply to be respected. One fears any inroad upon it, particularly during a period of moral decline.

The fact that the only government which allowed euthanasia was also one which indulged in both murder and genocide adds further fire to the opposition to euthanasia. This is regrettable because emotional outbursts about Nazis do not help rational debate.

The Case for Voluntary Euthanasia

A man should have the right to decide how much suffering he is prepared to accept.[306] When that limit is reached, it should be a basic human right for a man to lay down his life.[101] He may have used it well, finished all he started, be content to go, and have a terminal disease. Then follows what Lord Dawson described in the House of Lords in 1936 as a 'gap'. During this time life is useless to the man. His weakness increases gradually, attended by mounting suffering. He sees his family anxious and exhausted by nursing him. As Lord Dawson said,

... the shortening of the gap should not be denied when the need is there. This is due not to a diminution of courage, but rather to a truer conception of what life means and what the end of its usefulness deserves.

The sum of human suffering would be reduced by the introduction of voluntary euthanasia, so it must be a good measure, and this is why Plato and St Thomas More both advocated it.[130] And did not Jesus say, 'Greater love hath no man than this, that a man lay down his life for his friends' (John 15: 13; John 10: 18)?[402]

The fact that Christian ethics are traditionally opposed to euthanasia and suicide is irrelevant, since most of our modern society is not Christian. The minority who are have no right to impose their opinions on the whole nation.[306] Anyway, Christians are divided on the matter. Dean Inge of St Paul's said, 'I do not think we can assume that God wills the prolongation of torture for the benefit of the soul of the sufferer.'[391]

Doctors would soon come round to the idea when they realized that it lifted from their shoulders an agonizing decision.[361] They could apply all their techniques of re-suscitation until such time as the patient indicated that he had had enough: no longer need they worry about when to stop their treatments, or about people dying in great discomfort due to over-zealous treatment.[346] Further, when someone developed humiliating senile dementia, if he had signed the form previously, his family and the State could be relieved of the onerous duty of looking after him.[91]

It cannot be stressed enough that the proposal is only for *voluntary* euthanasia. A patient who wanted his life prolonged would be free to have it prolonged, and need not sign the form. No one would be brow-beaten into signing. No one would be killed who had not asked to be. No doctor or nurse who objected on grounds of conscience would be obliged to cooperate in the killing.

That, as well as I can put it, is the case *for* euthanasia, and while it is nonsense in my opinion, it is only fair to include these views.

Legal Considerations

I shall first consider the principles on which basic human rights depend, and then look at euthanasia in the context of these rights.

When Moses summarized his law, he gave ten commandments and did not mention rights at all. The English Common Law works in the same way, and yet we in this country rejoice in greater freedom than almost any other. Here is how Maitland explained the working of law in his *Constitutional History of England*: *

Now the great mass of our ordinary criminal law is made up of prohibitions, of the imposition of negative duties, its language is 'Thou shalt do no murder', 'Thou shalt not steal' and so forth. It does not say 'Thou shalt succour thy neighbour in distress' – I commit no crime by not pulling my neighbour out of the water, though thereby I could save his life without wetting my feet. So again our law as to civil injuries, 'Torts' as we call them, consists of prohibitions – I am not to assault or slander or defraud my neighbour, trespass on his land or damage his goods. Generally it takes some contract or some special relationship or some office to create an active duty. In the greater number of cases in which anyone is bound actively to do something, he is bound because he has agreed to be bound.

The secret which makes Magna Carta and Moses' Pentateuch great codes of law allowing considerable freedom to the men governed under them is their clear and precise statement of the duties of a citizen. I have rights because other men observe their duties, not the other way about. I have the right to walk the streets of England without let or hindrance only so long as no one attacks or robs me. If they do, of what value to me is my right? I have the right to a secure home until someone pillages it. If a

* Cambridge University Press, 1968, p. 501.

burglar or an official of customs and excise breaks in, where has my right gone? Rights follow from the observation of duties by the community. Therefore good laws tell a man his duties. Weak law speaks of his rights, and is almost unenforceable, because there has to be a court argument to prove that the injuring party is acting unconstitutionally. This involves weeks of legal wrangling, whereas it is easy to prove that someone has failed in a specific duty.

Any 'right to death' involves a corresponding duty to kill. To say there are conscience clauses in the Bill is no help.[255] As with abortion, the public would soon, quite correctly, be demanding euthanasia as a right, and putting pressure on dissenting doctors.

'Thou shalt do no murder' permits of no legal disputes, no governmental misapplication. It is a natural law. It states my duty. If the State exacts this duty from all, then I am safe; free to come and go, free from fear. My liberty is not curtailed by having to observe this duty towards others.

From what do such duties spring? Clearly they are universal. They are owed by the Prime Minister, the foreign visitor, the policeman, the Bishop, the Lord Mayor and me. They are owed to everyone and any exceptions have to be specially defined by specific laws (such as the Mental Health Act which permits a doctor to detain an insane man for his own and other people's safety). If the duties of a citizen are not observed, the result is a loss of freedom by the whole community. If I cannot make an aeroplane journey without danger of hi-jacking, if I cannot let my wife walk alone down the street at night, if my house can be broken into by the gas company because my bill was lost by the Post Office, if I fear that my doctor may kill me when I become a burden; then by so much is my freedom curtailed.[262] If I am less free, then so is the rest of the community.[80]

It is man's nature to live in communities, to trade, to work, to learn and teach. If a community is to enable the individual to grow, then he must be free. If there is to be freedom in any society, then basic duties must be fulfilled by all. It is evident, therefore, that the duties spring from the Nature of Man. They were not invented by Moses or King John's Barons. There are no communities in which they do not apply – anywhere on earth, any time in history. As Edmund Burke said:

> The principles that guide us, in public and in private, as they are not of our devising, but moulded into the nature and the essence of things, will endure with the sun and the moon – long, very long, after Whig and Tory, Stuart and Brunswick, and all such miserable bubbles and playthings of the hour, are vanished from existence and from memory.

Duties arise in many situations. If I hold a knife, I have a duty not to stab someone with it. If I borrow money, I have a duty to repay it. As I am a parent, it is my duty to feed my children. As I am a doctor, my duty is to restore my patients to health. Trade Unions have the duty to defend the rights of their members; it is the duty of Parliament to govern and defend the realm. Always it is something owed to the weaker by the stronger. In the natural order of things the men to whom we owe the most, the ones who receive most, are therefore the weakest, the poorest and the humblest. Is this not what civilization is all about? Nature requires of us that we provide our best care, our greatest concern, our strongest protection, for the infant and for the senile and dying, because they cannot help themselves.

To fail to provide for the needs of the dying is to fail in a basic duty. The self-evident requirements of a dying man are to have his symptoms relieved, and to be allowed to die with dignity and peace of mind. If we evade all the difficult problems he presents and just kill him, we have failed. Whether such euthanasia were voluntary or not is irrelevant: it is our duty so to care for these patients that they never ask for euthanasia. A patient who is longing to die is not being treated properly.[44] If we are not treating him properly, the solution is to improve our treatment, not to kill him. Is this not self-evident?

As it stood, Lord Raglan's Bill of 1969 gave inadequate definitions of who could and who could not request euthanasia. One does not, after all, want to make it easier for doctors to commit murder, or for depressed people to enlist assistance with suicide. But under the Bill a person could request to be killed if he had a 'serious physical illness or impairment reasonably thought in the patient's case to be incurable and expected to cause him severe distress or render him incapable of rational existence'.

Let us reflect on these provisions. It is simply not possible to decide which illnesses are physical and which mental. Senility, for instance, has a physical basis in impairment of blood flow to the brain by hardening of the arteries which supply it. The patient with heart disease in his fifties could say he had an incurable illness very likely to cause him distress. Distress is so subjective – do we accept the patient's assessment of whether it is severe or not? If so, how could one exclude arthritis, asthma, psoriasis or even schizophrenia? There is no way of telling whether a patient's depression is pathological or normal and reasonable in the circumstances. Where is the dividing line between rational and irrational existence?

All things considered, it would be hard to refuse anyone in late middle age and the Bill would have opened the door for death on demand. This may be what some of its advocates wanted, but I am sure it was not what the majority – including Lord Raglan – ever intended. The Bill was altogether unworkable, and Lord Raglan himself acknowledged this before retiring from the debate. He said in the London Medical Group conference on 5 February 1972 that he could not envisage any Bill with adequate safeguards, and that anyway euthanasia would be unnecessary if terminal care all over the country were brought up to the standard he had seen in the hospices. Such a retraction by an eminent person takes great courage, and we can only admire Lord Raglan's 'bold, just and impartial spirit'.

Had the Bill been passed into law, it would have been the one and only exception to the old legal principle that the consent of the victim is no defence for the infliction of an injury. (Assault, for instance, is no less a crime if the victim is a masochist and requested or enjoyed the assault.)[74] As I mentioned on page 130, surgical operations are justified by the legal doctrine of necessity, but euthanasia could not be. As Chancellor Garth Moore points out,* death for a man is, in the eyes of the law, a greater evil than pain, and so one could not say that a greater evil was averted by the deliberate killing of the patient.[20]

To admit into the Law the concept that some lives are not worth living would be very dangerous. As the Abortion Act has crystallized a cheapening of the popular respect for human life, so would the passing of a euthanasia Bill.[79] The risk of abuse would be high, and another bale of straw would be on the camel's back, the camel being civilization itself.

The precise definition of just which lives are not worth living has defeated the drafters of euthanasia legislation. The proposal to define any offence – such as the 'mercy killing' proposal of the Criminal Law Revision Committee – by the characteristics of the victim raises an important point of principle: is there really a case for assuming that some lives should be more terminable than others, that killing a human being in a defined category is less serious than killing a human being who is not in that category? An editorial in *The Times*[367] commented: 'The termination of a human life – whatever the physical or mental condition of that life – is a very grave matter. Its seriousness ought not to be minimized by an amendment of the law which, however well intentioned, could have the effect of making certain kinds of killing seem trivial.'

*p. 50 of 'Decisions about Life and Death' – Church Information Office – see Bibliography.

Medical Considerations

Mrs H. had a cancer of the womb. The surgeon was optimistic that he had successfully cured her, but a year later a lump could be felt again and she looked ill. Rapidly her abdomen swelled up and some fluid was removed from it. The diagnosis was obvious: the cancer had recurred and was so widespread that the abdominal lining was being irritated so that it exuded the fluid. She came to the hospice for terminal care. Every fortnight I relieved her abdominal distension by removing two or three gallons of fluid. She lost weight steadily. After several months the laboratory had been consistently unable to isolate malignant cells from the fluid, and Mrs H. was still not dead. We began to wonder about the diagnosis. Eventually the surgeon agreed to do a further operation to see what was happening. The operation had the air of a mystery tour. What we found was a gigantic cyst on the ovary which filled her entire abdomen. Her weight loss was due to the great quantity of protein she lost in the fluid I was removing.

Mrs H. is back at home leading a normal life.

What if the diagnosis of cancer (which made her depressed at first) had led to legal euthanasia? Mistaken diagnosis is a commonplace in medical practice.[43]

A lady who was sent to us with a brain tumour which had paralysed her right side had had an operation in which the surgeon had been unable to remove the growth. The diagnosis of a highly malignant 'astrocytoma' was confirmed by looking at a piece of it under a microscope. The tumour continued to grow, producing a big lump on the side of her head. Her paralysis spread, her speech and vision were lost and she became incontinent. Her weight increased to about 18 stones. Drowsiness developed and progressed to coma. For a month she made little response at all to the daily visits of her devoted young husband. Then the lump went down. She woke up. The power of speech returned, and her limbs began to move.

The physiotherapist set to work with delight, teaching her first to stand again, then to walk. The neurosurgeon assured me that her recovery could only be temporary. A year after she came to us, he saw her again, and expressed surprise to me that she was still alive. He embarked upon further investigations. To everyone's astonishment there was no sign whatever of the tumour. She was rehabilitated and is now home again, her only residual disability being blindness, with which she can cope.

But that is not all. When the hospice appeared on television, a conversation with this lady was broadcast. Several friends asked me 'who that wonderful girl was'. She radiated an amazing joyfulness to everyone she met. The other patients adored her; to be reminded of her is uplifting. Her illness seemed to have been tailor-made to teach her something of profoundest significance.

What if her loss of consciousness had led to legal euthanasia?

A few years ago a patient died of whom I was very fond. Mrs L. had spent a good half of her seventy-nine years, including most of her childhood, in hospitals because she was born with dislocated hips. Adequate treatment was not known in those days and severe arthritis developed. In addition a war injury had left her totally bedbound. The arthritis caused unending and sometimes severe pain. When I first knew her she never smiled, and always grumbled. The bed, the nurses, her tablets, the food, me – everything was wrong and she had innumerable minor complaints and symptoms. There was indigestion, sore mouth, severe itching, cataract in the eyes, sore throat, pain on movement, sinusitis and so on. On one occasion she said to me, 'I wish I was in me box', and no wonder. Then an eminent rheumatologist saw her, and while he said that nothing could be done for her arthritis that we were not already doing, he diagnosed chronic depression and suggested that we should treat that.

The treatment worked wonders and Mrs L. was urged to try some occupational therapy. Extra large needles that her deformed hands could grip were found, and some thick wool. She was cajoled into knitting me a scarf of prodigious length. It was followed by bedjackets, blankets, another scarf and finally an exquisite tea cosy incorporating four different colours of wool. This latter was presented to us as a wedding present by a beaming Mrs L. In fact she beamed at everyone and I found her surreptitiously reading a copy of *Lolita*. Not long before she died, I asked her if she still had pain. Her reply, after forty years of sulking, was astonishing: 'Oh yes, but it's no trouble.' There, finally laid aside, was the hang-up of a lifetime. Certainly it took other people's help; that's why the Almighty put more than one of us on the globe. But the great step forward was entirely her own. Wherever she is now, Mrs L. doesn't need her arthritis because she learned all it had to teach. This growing into a finer, bigger person is work, spiritual work, the most important work she had ever done.

What if her unrelieved pain had led to a legal euthanasia, as she had once suggested?

We admitted a Mr N. with a very painful cancer, profoundly depressed. His wife had reacted to his illness with an anxiety state and his three teenage sons with resentment. He was very cut off. Gradually the boys came to terms with his condition and with a new picture of their father. Now he was no longer at home, his wife calmed down, and the boys started visiting. They found a new respect for their father in spite of his physical deterioration. With help from nurses and social workers, the whole family gradually came together again.

Had he been euthanased because of pain (which we controlled, of course) this could never have happened, and the rejecting family who agreed to the killing would have felt very guilty afterwards. Guilt is a common concomitant of grief, especially if the dead person committed suicide. What would the misery be like, afterwards, for relatives who had consented to the killing of their kin?

A very unhappy old lady called Mrs E. came to our clinic at the hospice one Thursday. Her husband had just died. The grief had caused a flare-up of her arthritis. She was much weakened by a cancer. In tears she complained that life was not worth living. She didn't want to go on. Couldn't I just finish her off, please – that euthanasia thing she's seen them talking about on telly?

'You mean you want me to kill you?' I asked.

'Yes I do.'

'Well all right then,' I said reluctantly, 'There's no one would know, I suppose. Only me and the nurse – and she won't say anything, will you, Sister?' (Sister shot me an anxious look.) 'We'll do it now love, with an injection. Hold your arm out. Sister, pass me a syringe – no, not that. The big one. We'll need a lot to be sure to kill her. Come on, Mrs E. – hold your arm out.'

But the arm was behind her back. She gave a nervous giggle (Sister was looking quite demoralized). Then Mrs E. said something which I will never forget – 'No, doctor. What I mean is ... aren't you going to do something to *help* me?'

Of course we did help her, and Mrs E. lived to tell the story with some amusement to a TV interviewer several months later for a programme about the alternatives to euthanasia. What a lesson there was in her words. Just as, when a young person attempts suicide, we recognize it as a desperate cry for help, so ought we to begin to realize that the request of an old person for euthanasia is the same cry.

Are you cold? Are you lonely? Is your pain inadequately controlled? Never mind. I'll put all that right. I'll kill you.

What a response to human distress! We should be thankful none of the death brigade were around when men were struggling to conquer smallpox, cholera, TB, vagrancy and poverty in our society. A steady look at the problems of the dying or the elderly does not produce in the mind either the solution 'Kill them quickly' or 'Don't let them die!' These would both be opposites of neglect, certainly, but not the only alternatives.

If anyone really wants euthanasia, someone must have failed him.[93]

As I showed in the previous chapter, it is not the duty of a doctor to produce candidates for euthanasia by administering inappropriate treatment to the senile and dying. Neither is there any need for the shortening of their life. Properly cared for, the potential candidate for the euthanasiast's needle will find new meaning in this very important part of life – for dying is still a part of living. In this period a man may learn some of his life's most important lessons. As I hope the above examples show, the 'gap' of which Lord Dawson spoke (see p. 141) can be a very full one, and very productive.[23] Death need not be the final crushing defeat. On the contrary, a man can make a positive achievement of dying, a great final step forward.

Once a patient feels welcome, and not a burden to others; once his pain is controlled and other symptoms have been at least reduced to manageable proportions, then the cry for euthanasia disappears.[332] It is not that the question of euthanasia is right or wrong, desirable or repugnant, practical or unworkable. It is just that it is irrelevant. Proper care is the alternative to it, and will be universally available as soon as there is adequate instruction of medical students in our teaching hospitals.[72] If we fail in this duty to care let us not turn to the politicians asking them to extricate us from the mess.

Mr R., who was in a hospice for five weeks before he died, summed up the situation nicely: 'A few days before I came here,' he told me, 'the pain got so bad that I was afraid I would die. By the time I got here, I was afraid I wouldn't. But now I'm here, I'm glad I didn't!'

... a mind fixed and bent upon somewhat that is good doth avert the dolours of death. – Bacon[18]

Social Considerations

The innocent and the just thou shalt not kill. (Exodus 23:7)

The Jewish-Christian tradition has stated this law, not as a theoretical standard, but because it is a basic requirement for the cohesion of civilized society.

Because of a lack of caring in our community some people die in distress. The same lack of caring leads people to suggest euthanasia as a solution. People are lonely, miserable and in pain because no one has troubled to relieve them. Euthanasia is suggested as the solution because still no one troubles to care. It would be an attractive easy option.[133]

The patient who was driven to ask for euthanasia would not be alone with his decision. The substance of our lives is in relationships with others. We are dealing with an interlocking community, not with isolated individuals. It follows that a law for individual relief should not be introduced until its social consequences have justified it.

To pass legislation permitting even a small number of doctors to kill some of their patients would be to introduce a whole new image for the medical profession – that of licensed killers.[204] If it accepted the legalization of euthanasia, society would expect the medical profession to help it to avoid the agony of looking after people who are seriously ill. It would affect the community's attitude to compassionate and constructive care of the elderly. It is a significant fact that there have never been any geriatricians among the Voluntary Euthanasia Society's membership.

At present, when one is sick, the hypodermic needle or the pain-killing draught are welcomed as a means of relief. But suppose it were possible that the needle or draught were not for relief, but to kill? Could trust survive? Such legislation would bring pressures on the old and ill to get themselves out of the way. It would be like saying, 'If you cannot do anything you are worthless.' The most considerate people would be the ones to suffer most. Whether loved or not, many would feel it encumbent upon them to request euthanasia because they did not wish to be a trouble to their family and friends. What of the slightly confused or forgetful old person who was not quite sure whether she had signed the paper or not? What of the person whose family wanted to be rid of him, and said so?[276] Would you yourself not prefer euthanasia to going into some of the old folks' homes in this country *in their present state*?

Were good care not possible at all, one would have to consider drastic alternatives. But since it certainly is possible and working examples abound, our efforts must be directed towards improving the attitude of society to the old and dying. We must rediscover and reaffirm their role in community life.[244]

The Archbishop of Canterbury read the following from an eight-year-old's essay about grandmothers to the House of Lords: [146]

Grandmothers don't have to do anything but be there. They are old so they shouldn't play hard or run. They should never say 'hurry up'. Usually they are fat, but not too fat to tie children's shoes. They wear glasses and funny underwear, and they can take their teeth and gums off ... When they read to us, they don't skip bits or mind if it is the same story over again. Everybody should have one, especially if you don't have television, because *grandmothers are the only grown-ups who have time*. [My italics.]

If we prefer the alternative – killing people (whether they ask for it or not) – we must contemplate the practicalities. If many doctors declined to kill patients (as is the case with abortion) there would arise special nursing homes for the purpose, with a doctor's fee. What should we call them? Disposal units? Thanatoria?[63]

Consider the patient's relationships with his family. Usually no one would mention euthanasia or even death. But if they did, even from well-intentioned motives, a strain may be put on his relationships with them. Suppose a patient wanted euthanasia and his wife didn't agree (if she hid the signed form, Lord Raglan's Bill proposed a punishment of life imprisonment for her). Suppose half the family wanted the doctor to kill the patient and half did not. And what if a sister, say, discovered afterwards that the patient's wife had agreed. In short, would this legislation really reduce the sum of human suffering?

All things considered, do we really think that we have an improvement, in today's world, to replace our Christian moral code, our tradition of law and freedom, and our rich heritage of skill and knowledge? The principle of euthanasia, voluntary or involuntary, would run counter to Christian and Jewish morality; would limit our freedom by introducing a new fear for the elderly; and would misdirect the discoveries of science, which was properly intended for man's use in overcoming his adversities, not for evading them by instant death.

Even now the euthanasia lobbyists who are pressing for further discussions in Parliament are asking whether deformed children could not also be put to silence. Where will this end? Can an ancient and unbending moral law be superseded by what seems expedient and kind to well-meaning individuals? Where is the great Teacher who can redirect mankind into a better ethical code than that established by Christ, or Moses, or Buddha?[233]

If He is among the euthanasia lobby, let Him come and teach us.

Moral Considerations

> How long will ye give wrong judgement:
> and accept the persons of the ungodly?
> Defend the poor and fatherless:
> see that such as are in need and necessity have right.
> Deliver the outcast and poor:
> save them from the hand of the ungodly.
> They will not be learned nor understand,
> but walk on still in darkness:

all the foundations of the earth are out of course.
I have said, Ye are gods:
and ye are all the children of the most Highest.
But ye shall die like men:
and fall like one of the princes.

Psalm 82 : 2–7, *Books of Common Prayer*

However a man may appear, there is reflected within him the highest and finest principle in the universe (how else could he speak of unity, of justice, or of love?). It may be thickly covered over, but it cannot be extinguished. For this reason the Quakers say, 'There is that of God in every man.' That inner perfection can be served and respected in all men. There is no man who cannot receive love and be enriched by it. Good, sincere caring renders euthanasia unnecessary.

As the psalm suggests, it is man's nature to be immortal, constant and wise. The best law reflects these qualities. What the majority want is no basis for law. How can it be based on 'public opinion' which alters daily? Such ethics spring from expediency, which is shifting and unreliable. This is why the great law-givers of our history have been followed and respected: they provided a code based on eternal principles more in accord with the nature of man. Moses did not invent the Ten Commandments any more than did Newton the law of gravity. They both simply gave expression to laws inherent in Nature.

The greatest law-givers saw that the relaxation of the rule forbidding one man to kill another would lead to social decline. Lesser men, notably the Stoics,[109] subsequently made all manner of exceptions to the rule: for 'enemies', for criminals, for gladiators, for unborn babies, and finally, it is suggested, for the senile and suffering. All these exceptions are open to question. Society currently denies a man the 'right' to euthanasia in order to conserve wider freedoms.[388]

Even from the individual's point of view, one must consider what a request for euthanasia really means. Is he trying to escape, to get away with something? Perhaps it is not possible to evade justice (hence the Roman Catholic doctrine of purgatory, and the Buddhist teaching of re-incarnation and Karma). But usually the man who requests euthanasia is just uttering a cry for help and doesn't want to die at all, as I have shown. Should not any request for euthanasia alert us to reconsider the quality of our care for the person?

Suffering and death can never be eliminated from human experience, but the attitude of mind which wants to deny their existence and always to escape from them can be overcome. Man can grow bigger than his troubles. With help, any man can do this – it is not just for the rare saint. I looked after a building foreman, for instance, who died sitting in an armchair. He had firmly refused bed for weeks, in spite of considerable shortness of breath, because he just wouldn't give in – he wanted to watch all that happened in the ward. I was filled with admiration, and the other men in his ward were filled with confidence, by his example.

Frequently the advocates of euthanasia refer to a 'meaningless' or 'useless' life.[232] In my practical experience these descriptions can never be applied to human existence of any kind with certainty. No man is useless who can still receive love from others. No life is meaningless in which any measure of self-realization is still possible.[99]

When a nurse described to me how she cared for patients with brain damage, I was so impressed that I asked her to write down what she had seen.

As a very young inexperienced orthopaedic nurse I was sent to work in the annexe reserved for unconscious patients. Most of them had been severely injured in car accidents.

I 'specialed' three patients and consequently spent a great deal of time with them. What I remember most about the work was the amount and quality of love that these patients drew from me. It shocks me to think that some people would dismiss them as 'vegetables'. You can have no communication with a vegetable.

I worked mainly alone with them, except when their bed linen was changed, and I talked constantly to them. One patient in particular that I remember with a feeling of reverence, almost of awe, was called Jimmy. He was middle-aged, semiconscious and spastic. Jimmy was tube-fed and had a tracheostomy which needed frequent sucking out. I used to talk to him and put my finger over his tracheostomy to listen to his response. I used to talk to him about getting better as being just a matter of willpower, but I was mainly concerned to help him to communicate. I taught him to say 'yes' and I was acutely aware that he knew exactly what was going on and was making marathon efforts to communicate with me.

My memories of working with these patients leave me with a feeling of worship. Their silent presence had about it an atmosphere more akin to a cathedral than a greenhouse.

The use of this word 'vegetable' – or, even more repugnant, 'cabbage'[293] – is one of the most alarming degradations of modern medicine. An attempt to make it scientifically respectable – using the word 'vegetative' to describe the bodily functions of a decerebrate patient – is laughable.[440] What is scientific about it? Wherein does an unconscious man resemble a vegetable? Photosynthesis? Roots? Edibility? Science implies precise observation, confirmed by demonstration, leading to logical conclusions. I challenge anyone to demonstrate to me the vegetable attributes of a man.

As Dr Cicely Saunders said to a students' conference in 1974, 'A vegetable does not have relations and has no past.' There are many alternative terms to describe the damaged person – unconscious, decorticate, with only physical functions, decerebrate and so on. Such descriptions describe the lesion without questioning the patient's basic humanity.

An unconscious man has a body which breathes and has needs quite different from those of herbage, or those of animals. Even if the man is not there, the body is still the symbol of a man: the most sensitive and intelligent product of evolution yet to appear on Earth. It is a house which can be inhabited by a creature capable of contemplating Justice, Eternity and Truth. To the minds of other men this symbol is a very significant one. To violate it damages the mind and puts the social order at risk.

Indeed, before we can violate the integrity of a person we have mentally to demote him. So we invent a name which we can despise. It does not matter what the sub-human name is: its effect is to alter our attitude to the persons concerned. They become disposable.

The other dangerous thing about such terms is that they are imprecise. The word 'vegetable' began by being applied to people who were completely unresponsive. Then it was used for the very senile and for mentally defective babies. Now it is being used to describe perfectly rational people who are quadriplegic after accidents. Indeed, a lady who was able to write to the radio programme *Any Answers?* used the term to describe herself!

Applying this word to humans whose bodies are damaged or unconscious can change our whole willingness to care for and give to them of our best. Its use suits the euthanasia lobby well. Talk of killing people grates a bit, so one must justify it with obscuring terminology. I am not, of course, advocating intensive therapy for these unfortunate people to keep them alive indefinitely, but while they are alive I say that they, too, are worthy of respect. In their presence we should guard our tongues and be awake to their every need. Because they cannot communicate their needs, the nursing must be doubly good.

Use the right words and you can justify anything. Thinking can so easily be muddled. Take for example a letter to *The Times*, which the Rev. Dr Leslie Weatherhead wrote:

Those who condemn euthanasia on religious grounds seem to have lost their sense of logic. They say, 'leave it to God'. I would like to show them the parts of my garden that I have left to God! ... We are to cooperate with God by using all available human help and we are to use our common sense. Man seeks to be the master of birth. He must just as sensibly seek to be the master of death. I would willingly give a patient Holy Communion and then remain while a doctor took measures to allow the patient to slip into the next phase of being while some degree of dignity remained.[402]

A few days later a doctor replied:

A medically qualified person is not needed. After all, our hangmen – and most murderers – were and are not medically qualified. With short instruction, any reasonably intelligent person could do the final act. People with sufficient sense of responsibility, such as lawyers and parsons, could be trained and appointed legal thanatophores. Dr Weatherhead, for example, could administer Holy Communion, the Cup of Blessing, and then the *coup de grace*.[190]

The point to note in reply to Dr Weatherhead is of course that 'all available human help' for his garden would consist in pulling out the weeds of pain and despair, not blowing up the whole allotment.

10. Counselling the Dying

Oh why do people waste their breath
Inventing dainty names for death?

Sir John Betjeman, *Churchyards*

At his best, Man has no fear of death. The function of psychotherapy is simply to remind a man who he is. Our present-day conspiracy to ignore death looks like a community-sized act of cowardice. As Katharine Whitehorn said, 'Somehow we've got to get death back into the conversation, stop sheltering children from any faintest contact with it; work out what things we would die for, the things without which we would not care to go on living.'[412]

The main reason why communicating with patients about death is shirked is because it is painful to all concerned.[35] The family doctor is usually the most suitable person, if he is a trusted friend. People can put up with a great deal of discomfort if they are confident that those who are caring for them are concerned for their comfort, and respect them as individuals. Endless difficulties arise when a man has been deceived about his diagnosis. If he thinks he should be recovering, he may demand more active treatment when he finds he is getting weaker.[126] He may fail to put his affairs in order, or to consult his priest if he is a religious person. Suggestions of radical treatment may alarm him because he has never really faced the truth, although he probably suspects it. Half the fear of a serious prognosis may be a fear of suffering, sometimes quite bizarre, which can be allayed by reassurance and common sense.[252] If there is no frank discussion, this kind of fear can never be relieved. For the fears will almost certainly be there, made worse by uncertainty.

It is commonly supposed that if someone's fears that he may be dying are confirmed, he will go to pieces, turn his face to the wall and die. 'I can take it, but he couldn't,' relatives say, and if this is challenged they add 'I know him better than you do. It'd kill him.' In fact the response of deep depression and never coming out of it is rare.[404] People are thinking, 'How would *I* feel if I was given a death sentence for tomorrow?' and not considering the patient at all. To be asking questions about his illness and about dying, the patient must have been thinking about it for weeks. Before talking about it, he will nearly always have faced it and largely come to terms with it. There is no question of a sudden death sentence.

A doctor has not looked at his patients if he thinks they do not know when they are dying simply because he has not told them.[395] When relatives ask 'Do you think he knows?' we can point out that it is unlikely that he has not yet realized. 'After all,' I have said on occasions, 'he's not daft, is he?'[187] Surveys in hospitals by Professor Hinton[158] and Dr Exton-Smith[111] found a much higher proportion of patients with strong suspicions or actual knowledge of their diagnosis than had previously been believed.

There are so many ways that a patient can find out. He may read his hospital notes or overhear chance comments by relatives or doctors, or he may just draw the obvious conclusion when the family rally round, only to avoid him later because of their embarrassment.[226] One girl said to me, 'I knew it was cancer from the moment they started lying to me.'[360] Referral to a radiotherapy unit, or to a hospital known to specialize in cancer, is often seen by the patient as a death warrant, and should be discussed with him at once. People will never get to know that cancer can often be cured if they are never allowed to discuss it. Many people have declined to see their doctor with an early cancer because they have thought it might be incurable. All they need is to be assured that this view is now outdated.

When 231 people who were told that they had cancer were followed up in one survey,[4] only 7% said they would rather not have been told. One in five denied even having been told, which indicates that those not ready to know have a built-in defence against hearing. Certainly no harmful effects were recorded.[86] In a more recent survey Professor Hinton asked 60 patients with terminal cancer what they had been told.[160] Two thirds knew they were dying and none disapproved of open discussion. Nine were critical of the doctors and nurses for being evasive.

Of course a blunt stark thunderbolt is not the only alternative to telling lies.[195] The conversation should be led by the patient. The truth can be given in small doses over several meetings, and then in such a way that it does not hurt.[251] Here are a few examples of how the appropriate words come to mind when the actual situation presents itself:

Miss W. was in a slightly confused state, which added fears of madness to her fear of physical suffering. After several unsuccessful attempts to reassure her I said, 'Miss W., you're *all right*. You're just not immortal.' She relaxed and smiled. 'Good; I know,' she said, 'This is where the story ends.'

Mr T. asked if he had leukaemia. I said, 'No, nothing so awful as leukaemia, but trouble in the prostate gland.'

'I thought as much,' he said.

'Yes, it's acting malignantly, but obviously not very malignantly as you can see from the length of time you've had it.' (Over four years.) He looked relieved and went on to ask about his hearing aid.

Two days before Mr V. died we had this conversation, which said all that was needed without dredging up the hard words:

'They told me there was a shadow in my lung on the X-ray. What was it?'

'A bit of a growth on this side.'

'But they told me there was nothing to worry about.'

'There never is.'

'Good.'

Mr S. was a patient who wanted to leave everything to us, and made it plain that he did not want to know his diagnosis. I accepted this decision, but would not join in his imaginary game of 'when I get better'.

'Right,' I said, 'we'll get that pain of yours under control.'

'I'm glad of that. I'm not going to peg out just yet then?'

At first I hesitated (which he did not notice) before replying, 'Not *just* yet.'

'Oh good,' he said, 'I've got a lot of gardening to do.'

'Well, I'm not sure you'll be able to do very much of that.'

'No, I see. But I'll be able to potter about a bit?'

'We'll have to see how you go over these next few days.'

'All right. I'm glad you can do something for me.'

'Yes, we'll get rid of that pain.'

The point is that you give the patient a choice of directions for the conversation to take. He will indicate what he is ready to hear. It is almost like a dance. A man like Mr S. will come very gradually round to a fuller realization of his situation, at his own speed.

One patient wrote down for us his experience of being told his diagnosis of cancer. Here is what he said:

I had always had a subconscious dread of surgery, so that when I went for the first consultation I was apprehensive to say the least. But the surgeon was so forthright that when an operation was discussed, I felt such complete confidence in him that this banished all sense of fear.

I was admitted to hospital and very soon had the 'exploratory' operation. The following day I was told of the tumour in the gullet and that a major operation was essential. Again, because I was given the details of what was to be done, I felt no fear.

After the immediate post-operative discomfort I still had

difficulty with swallowing, and this caused me some depression. However, eventually I began to manage to swallow small quantities of soft food and by the time I was discharged my confidence returned. In the following weeks I appeared to make remarkable strides towards recovery and I began to plan the early return to various activities.

But then I began to feel my strength failing and my ambitions seemed less attractive – depression returned.

Then came the visits from the Out-Patients Sister* and the invitation to attend the Clinic. Soon I began to feel a new interest and visits to the Clinic became something to anticipate with real pleasure and the treatment soon brought about improvement.

Meantime a germ of suspicion had been forming in my mind that there might be something more than the weakness following a major operation, and I made some probing observations in the family to see if they were keeping something from me. I learned nothing!

Eventually I made up my mind – I would ask the direct question of the doctor. He had apparently come to a similar conclusion – I was now ready to be told.

I felt no sense of shock nor any fear – the doctor had crystallized my own thoughts and a feeling of calm and relief took the place of the doubt.

I am sure that in my weak and confused condition just after the operation and the depression of the ensuing weeks, it would have been quite wrong to burden my mind with the knowledge that I could not be cured.

After he had been told he was dying, this patient's wife wrote:

He took it very well – as I knew he would – and I now consider that it was right to wait until he regained his composure before revealing the facts. We are now able to discuss the future without difficulty and to make arrangements accordingly.

Other similar papers written by dying patients about their own plight are also revealing.[98]

Miss K., a Polish music teacher who knew that she was

* From a hospice.

dying, commented one day on her weakness and drowsiness. The conversation developed as follows:

'The weakness is due to your anaemia.'

'Aren't the tablets dealing with that?'

'They will help, but they can't really stop it. If we were to replace the lost blood by a blood transfusion into your arm, that would bring it back to normal. Would you like that?'

'What would happen then? Would I be cured?'

'Oh no. It would make you feel better, but you would have to go through the same process once more as the anaemia developed again. But it would mean that you would live a little longer.'

'I think I would prefer to be left in peace ... I am not afraid to die,' Miss K. continued, 'and I thank you very much, doctor, for giving me this warning, for taking the first step in preparing me for the long journey ahead.' When I left her, she was looking ... joyful? imperial? anyway, quite awesome. Her peace and strength never faltered until she died six weeks later.

Miss K. was well prepared to die, but in general people pretend that no such thing could ever happen, and they will need to be brought to acceptance gradually. Metropolitan Anthony (Archbishop Anthony Bloom) described his dismay and horror at the prevalent attitude to death which he found on coming to England:

I belong to a nation and to a Church [Russian Orthodox] where death is considered as part of life. Death is a normal thing – a function of man to face – and one of the things I met in this country is that death is almost an indecency. People shouldn't do that to their friends! And if they fall so low as to do it, generally one turns to specialists who can deal with the problem. That is, the dead person is left in a corner until the undertakers come and do what is to be done, after which the family and friends at best are confronted with the coffin . . .[36]

It is fascinating to notice how different people come to

accept death. A Mrs L., three weeks before she died, became suspicious of her failure to recover:

'I'm not making any headway, am I?'

'Not at the moment,' I said.

'When I had the operation for the cancer in my stomach
... I suppose it was a cancer, wasn't it ...?'

'Yes.'

'... I wonder if they left a bit behind?'

'It could be connected with that.'

'So I'll have to grin and bear it.'

For some days Mrs L. was difficult to nurse and then
declared that as we could do nothing for her, she was
going home. Her family came to us in panic – there was
no one to nurse her at home, how could she go? She
sullenly listened to me as I tried to reason with her, and
finally agreed to sleep on it. The next day a completely
different Mrs L. greeted me with a grin and said, 'All
right, I've settled.' She was cheerful for the whole of her
last week.

A dour Irish labourer, Mr D., made his peace with
death in a way that disrupted a whole ward. When he
found out that he was dying, he went into a huff and refused all medicines. He assailed me one morning with:

'Doctor! This is unsufferable.'

'Why?'

'It's very painful. Couldn't I be examined at the London
Hospital again?'

'There's nothing anyone can do to heal it, I'm afraid.'

'I want to see a specialist.'

'You already have, and he sent you to us. If you have
pain, it's your own fault; you refused the medicine.'

'I'm having no more medicine.'

'Then you'll have pain.'

'There's gin in the medicine,' interjected Sister, offering him the analgesic mixture. He wavered a moment,
then drank it with gusto, raising the glass aristocratically.

'They told me it was a widespread cancer,' he said.

'Yes,' I confirmed.

'So I'm not long here? Soon I'll be up there. And I'm ready to go.' (Raising his voice) 'Death where is thy sting? GRAVE WHERE IS THY VICTORY?'

I retreated.

In all such conversations the patient leads the way. The achievement is his, and the role of the caring team is only to watch for impediments which may disturb his peace of mind. Some will never come to terms with their fate, demanding reassurance to the last. 'They must be allowed their choice. They find their own way through and it seems clear to me that one does not necessarily have to know that death is imminent to be well prepared to meet it. Trust and faith in life and in death are not so very different.'[335]

Mr H. was a patient who made it clear that no further discussion would be appropriate. On arrival at the hospice, he said to me, 'As far as I know I've been sent here for convalescence. That's as far as I know.' Clearly he *did* know that he was very ill, but was not yet ready to face the fact.

It is not a case of what to tell a patient, but of what we will let him tell us.[326] We must just listen. Then the patient will give all the cues, however brief the conversation. When that little probing half-question comes up – 'That lump's bigger, isn't it?; I think the paralysis is spreading, nurse: I can't hold my cup these days'; and such like – when the question comes up – then we can be ready to recognize it and give a few minutes of honest listening. Tiredness, overwork or being in a rush can never be an excuse for refusing to give this inestimable help. If we really listen, then these little conversations do not usually take long, for time is not a question of length, it is a question of depth.

Even when dying, a person can still have a sense of purpose and self-esteem. The mode of dying will be as individual as the person himself. I even knew one old lady who told us the date of her death a week in advance. She had been told in a dream that she would meet her dead sister again on Friday the thirteenth. On the twelfth she looked so well that we joked about it, but the next day, having deteriorated suddenly, she announced that she would soon die. And she did.

A Mr D. wondered if he would reach his next birthday which was three weeks away.[49] 'Yes,' I said, 'but not the next one.' He smiled and said 'Good: I don't want to.'

A Mrs G. said to a hospice doctor, 'I'm getting weaker. Can't you do anything about it?'

'Not at the moment,' he replied.

'So I shall just get weaker and weaker?'

'You could also get happier and happier.'

'I know.' She smiled and relaxed: 'I've had a happy life.'

In this way a person's whole attitude can be deftly turned to bring out what is positive in them. However, it is not always such plain sailing, and some patients will need more of the counsellor's time. If we are to help, we first need to realize that seriously ill patients *will* have considered the possibility of death.[70] Professor Hinton found that nearly three quarters of a group of dying patients had a good idea that they were dying. Of those, one quarter thought that they might possibly die, a half thought that they were probably dying, and the rest knew that they were.[159]

This failure to communicate is largely a failure to listen, which is itself the principal therapy. Patients may experience a great relief just from being able to unburden themselves of fears, grief, feelings of guilt and failure, of loneliness or of frustration at being so dependent on others.[48] Sharing such feelings can be consoling for the patient, though rather uncomfortable for the listener. To render this service, we have to be prepared to be disturbed. By listening to a patient one can redirect his attention from his symptoms or worries, on to the topic being discussed. Alternatively one might enable him to bring some of his worst fears and suspicions out into the light of consciousness, where they will lose much of their strength. Emotions seen and understood are manageable, particularly if the patient can be reassured that they are not his guilty secrets but the sort of thing everyone feels in such circumstances. Fear that there will be pain can be countered with confidence.

The value of the companionship of a listener to dying people is delightfully described in a letter written by the philosopher Epictetus on the day of his death:

On this truly happy day of my life, as I am at the point of death, I write this to you. The diseases in my bladder and stomach are pursuing their course, lacking nothing of their usual severity; but against all this is the joy in my heart at the recollection of my conversation with you.

Sometimes there will be very little to be said. Mrs K., a doughty old Cockney, countered my probing questions with 'I know I've got something wrong with me,' and changed the subject. Just before she died, with the family all sitting around the bed, she fixed me severely with her eye and said, 'I'm just going to sleep, that's all.'

Denial, Dependence, Transference and Regression

The first thing people do with bad news is to sweep it under the carpet.

Mr L., a young family man with cancer of the rectum, said to me, 'Cor, this pain's killing me. Can't you do something about it?'

'Yes,' I said, 'we can control the pain.'

'Oh good, because my little lad's coming in this afternoon, and I don't want him to see me in this state. Blimey.'

Sometime later, after an injection of diamorphine, Mr L. asked me how long he would be in the hospice.

'I don't want to be off work too long. That injection did the trick. Thanks very much. I feel I could get up now – will that be all right? I don't want the family to think I'm bedbound!'

Despite severe pelvic pain and considerable loss of weight, Mr L. had returned to work after an exploratory operation and now felt extremely ill. His refusal to come to terms with his illness was cutting him off from everyone. The wall of optimism which he strenuously erected around himself made sympathy difficult, especially when he never even waited for answers to his questions. That he was obviously fearful of possible answers showed that subconsciously he knew his prognosis, but he was certainly not yet able to receive the concrete confirmation of his fears. Indeed, we had one lady with us who asked her diagnosis on three separate ward rounds, and each time denied having been told before; such was her refusal to face what she well knew. Because we meet this situation so frequently we have come to regard it as a normal development. This wall of denial is like the battlements of a medieval castle, where guards are ever vigilant, protecting the person until the moment when he is ready to face the truth.

'My wife's dead, most of my friends are dead, there's nothing left to hold me. I wouldn't mind if I were to die tomorrow.' This more aged patient spoke for the majority of his generation. They are usually willing to go.[425] But a few have difficulty with adjusting to the situation, and may need more skilled counselling.

A relatively common reaction when a person first begins to realize that a cure is not possible is anger. Quite a simple idea may be at the root of it, such as 'How dare my body let me down?' or 'Why can't this doctor stop playing about, and heal me?' or 'But I *must* look after the children until they have left school.' If the patient is very polite it may all come to the surface as an anxiety state, but usually he will direct the anger against some particular person or hospital. The counsellor can help him to see what the anger is really about, always bearing in mind that some of it may be quite justified. The most valuable help at such a time is a stable reliable person who can ride the storm – a 'father figure' as the jargon has it. The person usually most fitted for this role is the family doctor, though problems arise if the patient needs him, but is seen instead by a relief service doctor. The presence of such a supporting person, or group of people, brings the patient a great sense of safety.

It is part of man's nature to live in families. Throughout our lives our relationships with others reflect the original relationships in our early family life. In emotionally charged situations we may 'transfer' the full strength of our feelings of love or repulsion for childhood companions to the people caring for us. Criticism of, and undue involvement with, the patient can often be avoided if the staff understand this. Occasionally it helps the patient to be given some insight into these reactions. Only a skilled counsellor should embark on this, however, lest some precious relationship be upset when there is not time enough for the patient to rebuild it. The intensity of this transference of feelings is likely to be directed at the counsellor himself, and so Professor Cramond[70] stressed that the same counsellor should support the patient through to the end, otherwise the patient may suffer an additional bereavement.

When a newly-bereaved relative transfers his affection for the dead person on to one of the attendants who were caring for the family, and suddenly falls madly in love with a doctor or nurse, this can be one of the most embarrassing of all professional hazards. It is advisable to refer such occurrences to an experienced counsellor lest everyone gets hurt.

Another series of reactions which may be set off can be particularly exasperating for the nurses. It is called 'regression'. As more and more has to be done for the patient he becomes as dependent as a baby. Understandably his behaviour may become correspondingly childish. He may thus be defiant and rebellious in an effort to reassert his lost independence, or annoyingly demanding. The staff tend to reject such a patient, which makes him all the worse, or they may be mothering and indulgent, which an intelligent patient will resent.

Mrs G., for instance, a lady of seventy-seven with cancer of the tongue which had spread to the glands in her neck, asked me one day: 'What's this lump in my neck?'

'It's just the same as the one on your tongue,' I replied evasively.

'Whatever that is,' she parried, 'I know you won't tell me.'

'Of course I will, if you want me to.'

'What is it then? It is a cancer isn't it?'

'Yes, but it's all confined to this small area.'

'I've asked before several times,' she said. 'I told them I was old enough to know! ... Thank you. I'll just keep smiling and put up with it then.' Whereupon she smiled, splendidly.

Some people, in coming to terms with a grave prognosis, try to bargain for time. One man who said he wanted to put his affairs in order asked me his diagnosis. 'It won't upset me,' he said, 'whatever you tell me.' The word cancer was not used, but he was told his body was wearing out fast and would never be strong again. He asked how long he had left. I said I did not know, but it was probably only a few months. 'But I might hang on for a couple of years perhaps, would you say?' He said he would be willing to die, provided he could just have a holiday in the country first. In fact it is never advisable to give a prognosis of so many days, weeks or months that a patient will live. It will only be inaccurate and lay the prophet open to derision.[283]

Another patient asked each member of the medical staff what his prognosis was, trying to find someone who would make a lengthy forecast. Three days before he died, however, there was a total change. He compared dying to going to a new school – 'an alarming change, but pleasant in retrospect!'

Many people respond to the knowledge of impending

173

death with depression, particularly when they have pain which has not been properly controlled. Endless meaningless pain wears a person down, 'weakens his ego' as the saying goes, because there is no appropriate response to it, no apparent meaning in it. A counsellor may help the patient to discover a meaning in his suffering – something meaningful to the patient, that is, not necessarily to the counsellor – and as Dr LeShan says,

> It is perhaps important for the therapist first to be clear about his own feelings in this area before he can effectively help the sufferer. If he believes that there is a meaning, even if he cannot find it, he is in a much better position to help.[214]

I have a friend with multiple sclerosis with which he copes admirably, using a wheelchair and Possum typewriter. He frequently meets people as ill as himself or worse, and is a constant source of encouragement to them because they see how one man copes with overwhelming problems. He sees this as his role, and thus wrests advantages out of the disease itself.

A depressed patient will worry about unfinished jobs in the past or anticipated suffering and bereavement in the future. He can be reassured by stressing what he did achieve, what his life has stood for, and by being told that death will be peaceful. Indeed, if he is in a hospice with other dying patients he will see this for himself. If he feels that he is a nuisance to others at home, he can be told that his family really want him there. If he is in hospital it can be pointed out to him that the nurses and doctors only chose their kind of work because they wanted to help nuisances. However, guilty feelings should not all be dismissed and reassured away, even if that were possible. Guilt, and any pain or other 'conversion symptom' to which it gives rise, may be felt by a patient to be an atonement, a penance; without it he may feel that his values have gone, leaving him aimless. To quote Dr LeShan's paper again:

> The question should be asked. 'Is there a purpose behind

this pain in this particular patient?' 'Does it hold off guilt?' 'Does it provide him with a sense of being real that he desperately needs?' 'Is it a conversion symptom and, if so, of what?' One ignores these questions at the risk of successfully answering the patient's conscious plea for relief and destroying his adjustment.

None of these moods and attitudes will be fixed. If one looks afresh at a patient during each visit, he will be seen to fluctuate between being dignified and capable, and childishly dependent. He may behave regressively while being bathed, but responsibly when writing his will. If his dignity is to be maintained, some means of formally expressing his independence should be provided. He may be able to share in the doctor's decisions about his treatment; if he is capable of making things in occupational therapy, an opportunity should be provided for him to sell these to help provide for his family or to give to charity. Any 'when necessary' drugs could be given into his care; he could choose his meals from a daily menu, and keep his own photographs, ornaments or cards on a bedside locker so that his bed area bears the distinct stamp of his personality.[249] As long as he is able to, a dying man should manage his own affairs and be consulted on family problems. A policy of 'don't trouble him with that now, he's ill' will only worsen his feelings of isolation.

Some sort of support system is essential to deal with problems which arise as a patient swings between being dependent and self-sufficient. The person who gives this support should not usually be the one who does the nursing and the cooking, because this will only accentuate his dependent status. A complete outsider is more suitable, preferably a social worker, district nurse or psychiatrist. His visits can also provide support for the caring team as well as the patient, especially if rebellion in a patient is being projected on to other people or the institution caring for him. The staff can share with the counsellor any feelings of aggression towards a patient, or of bereavement if a favourite one dies.

These various patterns of interaction between people, and between patients and their environment, can give rise to difficulties which can be very absorbing to treat. They are, however, only mechanical malfunctions of the mind, and no more a substitute for the man himself than his body is. It is easy to suppose that, having mastered psychology, one has understood Man; but there is much more to see than these paintings on his shell.

While a head full of theoretical psychology can be of help in sorting out frankly pathological behaviour, it can sometimes get in the way of normal human communication. Attempts to 'understand' meaning 'classify under headings' just get in the way of listening. *Any* idea between the two people will get in the way. The most destructive ones are selfish thoughts: '*I* know exactly what he is talking about'; '*I* wish *I* understood these situations'; '*I* wish he hadn't asked *me*'; 'Am *I* giving anything away on *my* face?'; 'What did *I* say last time *I* was in this corner?'; 'What did *I* read in that book?' It is quite usual, when a patient asks a searching question, for people to root around for replies in the darkness in their own heads. There they find ignorance. For ignorance means ignoring. Ignoring what? Ignoring the one and only possible source of information which could tell us what to say to this patient, now. In the head of every one of us is a superb computer – to our knowledge the best yet to appear on this planet – which does know the right, the kind, the helpful answer to every need presented to us. But no computer can function correctly if the wrong information is fed into it. Only in this patient's voice and on his face at this moment are his present needs clearly expressed. If we STOP thinking and turn attention wholly out, hungrily, for that information, we can – all of us – utterly trust the computer to produce the answers. (If you *won't* trust this knowledge, go and watch television or something where you won't be in the way of useful people.) Now if the mind produces nothing at all to say, that also is reliable. In any difficult conversation, silences are in order. They are rests, not awkward silences, provided the attention is firmly kept off one's self on to the other person's needs. The chances are that the patient has not really expressed his deep question yet and is trying to find the words. And when you do speak, trust that you know what to say, letting it come without taking the attention back to yourself, because the computer still needs its data input. You might have to change direction in mid-sentence.

Support at the End

The dying need regular and frequent visits to show that interest is still being taken in them. Above all they must be assured that whatever happens they will not be deserted. At least one of the team should be with the family to support them throughout the terminal period, otherwise they will have no one in whom to place their confidence. This can be the social worker,[78] nurse[239] or family doctor.[56] If this person calls while the patient is asleep, he should at least leave a note to say that he has called.

The patient should be helped not to put things off 'until I feel better', and not to hold back from emotional contact with others on the same pretext.[212] He may need to be reassured that the end will not be long now, and that someone will be with him at the hour of his death.

I have known several who wanted to talk only a few hours before they died. They were not frightened nor unwilling to go, for by then they were too far away to want to come back. They were conscious of leaving weakness and exhaustion rather than life and its activities. They no longer had any pain but felt intensely weary. They wanted to say goobye to those they loved but were not torn with longing to stay with them. – Dr Cicely Saunders in *Care of the Dying* – see Bibliography

Finally we should remember that, since dying is a unique experience in each life, the man who is dying rightly expects some special consideration and indulgence.[271] Even those of us who see dozens of people die need to remember that what is familiar for us is for the patient his biggest adventure.

11. Grief

�֎

They that love beyond the world cannot be separated by it. Death cannot kill what never dies. Nor can spirits ever be divided, they love and live in the same divine principle; the root and record of their friendship. – From *Union of Friends* by William Penn

Part of care of the dying is care of the bereaved: they are two sides of the same coin.

It is important to understand that grief begins from the moment when a member of the family is told that the patient will not recover. As soon as a person realizes that a part of his life is soon to be torn away, a long process of grief begins which develops in recognizable stages. As a process of healing and replacement, it has been observed to involve work which the bereaved person has to do on himself. Other people can help, but there is no avoiding or sidestepping the process. As Helen Deutsch expressed it, 'the process of mourning as reaction to the real loss of a loved person must be carried to completion'[83] and some authorities consider that this applies even if the grief is suppressed or delayed by sedatives.

Research into bereavement is still in its infancy and many questions, particularly in relation to bereaved children, are still unanswered. There is controversy over many of the points mentioned in this chapter. All I can do is to present the findings and theories of a few prominent workers in the field.

The effort involved in grieving has been divided into

'worry work' before the loved person dies, and 'grief work' afterwards.[178] The way some of this work can be done before the death could be clearly seen in the parents of a teenager who died with us some years ago. They spent all their spare time with him in the ward, alert to his every need, fussing the nurses, questioning the doctors. His mother adjusted his pillows, straightened his sheets, tidied his locker and made him drinks almost incessantly. His father would show us photographs of the boy just before his illness had disfigured him. 'This is the real Dick,' he would say. 'This is how he really looks.' These parents were thus much more ready for the death when it came than they would have been had they not started grieving beforehand, though of course when the end came it was still a crushing experience for them.

Another couple took home a brother with a brain tumour so that his care could be supervised by the outpatients department of the hospice. The sitting-room became a sick bay, and the other members of the family took turns in sitting with him at nights. They devised ways of enabling him to sit up and eat in spite of paralysis, and of communicating when he lost the power of speech. As he lapsed into unconsciousness they began to give away his various treasures and handicrafts, as if parting from him bit by bit.

The way in which grief begins before the death was described by a man who knew his wife would never leave the hospice. 'It's like a desert at home without her,' he said. For this reason, no relatives should be told of a grave prognosis and then left to their own devices: they should at the same time be invited to come back and talk over their distress and questions. They will have so many decisions to make: Who should tell the patient that he is dying, and when? Should his house be sold? Should his son be recalled from Australia? How can he be asked to write a will? and so on. If the relatives are very upset and disorganized, they should be given something positive to do for the patient. For instance, they could be taught nursing procedures, or help with bathing or feeding a very weak patient.[350] This approach also helps people to get over the feelings of guilt which are often a part of grieving, as I shall explain later. Other relatives should be involved as much as possible, for it is the whole family which is bereaved, and together they can face it much better than each could alone.

Often a family will look for a scapegoat to blame for their misfortune. They may be angry – with God, with the hospital or with the individual members of the caring team. Doctors and nurses have to learn to accept this hostility without reacting. Arguing is no help: what is needed is understanding and a willingness to share their burden of misery. This is possible if they are simply encouraged to talk and then listened to carefully. Often a clergyman is the best person for this kind of support, and should be introduced to the family as early as possible in the course of the patient's terminal illness. As far as being angry with God is concerned, I will never forget the response of Dr Elisabeth Kübler-Ross to a patient who expressed guilt at such anger – 'Don't vorry. God can take it!'

Gradually the time will approach for saying goodbye, which should not be omitted. One husband confided, 'I know she must be worrying about me but she doesn't talk of it. I would so much like to tell her that I will manage when she is gone.' In this particular case the staff were able to break the ice for the couple, enabling them to share all their fears and hopes.

As the last hours approach, relatives may feel lonely. They will probably want to spend a lot of time with the patient, yet will need frequent attention and reassurance themselves. Comfortable chairs at the bedside, drinks and even meals should be provided. If they are obviously tired it can be suggested that they go and get some rest – in an adjoining room if possible. Some will want to be with the patient at the moment of death, others would prefer not to be. Neither course should be favoured or criticized by the staff, but rather reinforced by assurance that it is the right course for them, and by affording them every help. It helps if they can be given some idea of how soon the death will come, what the medicines or injections are for, and if they are told that the staff will not allow any suffering to disturb the patient's sleep.

When the death does occur, it will be a shock for the relatives, however well prepared they may be. One of the most helpful people at this point may be the undertaker,* getting on with his arrangements with quiet sympathy. But the relatives will need skilled support for much longer than he can offer it. When someone dies in hospital, therefore, the family doctor and the parish priest should be informed at once, so that they can mobilize help, particularly if the bereaved person has been left living alone. The family doctor should visit frequently[3] and the clergyman should call in during the second week after the bereavement, and then periodically over the first year. A social worker should also be brought in to advise on the handling of insurance claims, death grants, widow's pensions, deeds of probate and so on.

Normal grief generally proceeds through a series of predictable stages, though each individual will work through his own variation of the pattern.[39]

At first, for a few days, only occasionally for more than a week, the person behaves almost as if nothing has happened. He handles day to day affairs like an automaton, feeling numb and empty. One lady whose mother had just died was stopped by a neighbour on the street.

'Good morning, E., how's your mother?'

'Oh, she's fine, thanks,' came the reply, with a vacant smile.

After this numbness the pangs of grief begin. It is as though the person denies the fact of death to himself, and experiences intense yearning to be reunited with the dead person.[280] The mind searches for the lost companion, only to be painfully frustrated again and again. These feelings

* Mortician in the USA.

are all the more violent if the death was sudden and un-expected so that no proper 'worry-work' could be done.[178]

Dr Erich Lindemann described such pangs as

distress occurring in waves lasting from twenty minutes to an hour at a time, a feeling of tightness in the throat, choking with shortness of breath, need for sighing and an empty feeling in the abdomen, lack of muscular power, and an intense subjective distress described as tension or mental pain.[219]

Between these attacks

the bereaved person is depressed and apathetic with a sense of futility. Associated symptoms are insomnia, anorexia, restless-ness, irritability with occasional outbursts of anger directed against others or the self, and preoccupation with thoughts of the deceased. The dead person is commonly felt to be present and there is a tendency to think of him as if he was still alive and to idealize his memory. The intensity of these features begins to decline after one to six weeks and is minimal by six months, although for several years occasional brief periods of yearning and depression may be precipitated by reminders of the loss.[278]

Illusions of the presence of the dead person are common and normal, and may continue to occur at intervals for a decade or so. Some 50% of bereaved people in a Welsh study experienced these illusions of a dead spouse, and in Japan 90% of people did.[311] He may be seen sitting in his accustomed place, or heard to call the person's name, or to come in through the front door at the accustomed time each day. These experiences have also been recorded when the person is only thought to be dead, but in fact turns up again later, as happened frequently with prisoners of war for instance. It is therefore unlikely that they represent any real ongoing relationship with the dead. Nevertheless these visions can be shatteringly realistic, with all the power of a real meeting, because they may reveal some aspect of the dead person's personality which had been imperfectly observed during life and only emerges on reflection.

Since these phenomena spring from an inner denial of the death, and may be beautiful and revealing as often as frightening, they are to some extent treasured by the person experiencing them. If others try to comfort him, thereby implying confirmation of the death, their efforts may be resented. Dr John Bowlby says:

Thus, we see, repeated disappointment, weeping, anger, accusation and ingratitude are all features of the first phase of mourning and are to be understood as expressions of the urge to recover the lost object.*[39]

If a doctor has to ask for permission to perform an autopsy, he should remember that the bereaved person will probably be in the state described above, and consenting could feel to him like agreeing to the cutting up of a living person.

The pangs of grief gradually give way to depression and despair as the person unlearns the habits he has woven around the relationship with the deceased. The waves of grief lessen in frequency and intensity. Commonly a watershed occurs after about two years. Appetite and pride in appearance return and a new life is constructed. It is usually said that the process of adjustment is easier for the elderly, who expect death to come to their dearest, but for the young widow or parent it is harder.

Good general advice for the bereaved, particularly in countries whose traditions derive from Britain, is 'Don't try to be too wonderful. Let other people help you.'

To be able to counsel the bereaved effectively, the counsellor himself needs to see death as a meaningful event. He must talk frankly with grieving people, both during the period before the death and afterwards. In his book *Bereavement* (see Bibliography) Dr Colin Murray Parkes points out that:

*Dr Bowlby is not being callous in referring to someone a person loves as an 'object': it is an expression – albeit an ugly one – used regularly by psychologists.

pain is inevitable in such a case and cannot be avoided. It stems from the awareness of both parties that neither can give the other what he wants. The helper cannot bring back the person who is dead and the bereaved person cannot gratify the helper by seeming helped. No wonder that both feel dissatisfied with the encounter.

During the period of numbness and also during the early phase of the acute pangs of grief, bereaved people need help with almost everything, and especially with decisions. They need mothering. Hence the Jewish custom for the whole family to rally round the household during the period of 'Shiva' (seven days). Running the house and the funeral is not the duty of the dead person's nearest and dearest: they need very practical help; sympathy can come later, in the form of tolerance of the depression and irritability which may afflict the bereaved for several months. If you wish to visit Jewish friends during this period, you will find you are not intruding, but usually welcome. Ask which days they are 'sitting' (special low chairs are borrowed from the synagogue for the purpose). Men should take a hat and may enter the room if formal prayers are in progress. During these the ladies stay in the background in silence, or gather in another room and talk, talk, TALK.

The helpers should do nothing which will discourage the expression of appropriate grief. They should make it clear to the grieving person that they do not mind if he weeps. Over the next few weeks visits from friends will be appreciated, even if they are awkward occasions. The friends may find that they have to share some of the pain, to reassure the grieving person that his disorganization is normal and not a sign that he is going mad. Any mention of suicide, however, should be taken seriously and is an indication for referral to a psychiatrist or skilled social worker for help.

In a hospice there are often a number of bereaved people who are working through their grief by doing voluntary work for a few months following the death. The best help for the grieving, however, comes from other people who are in the same situation. Bereaved mothers or widows are more likely to find support from other parents or widows similarly stricken than they are within their own families.[81] A local clergyman can often bring together a group of widows for self-help, and there are two organizations which are rapidly becoming nationally important in this field. 'Cruse',* founded in 1959 by Margaret Torrie, gives practical and friendly advice and help to widows and their children by the provision of information sheets and by direct counselling on a local or national level.

Though Cruse clubs are social clubs in several parts of the country, the main function of the national organization is not to provide social support but a counselling service to widows, particularly those in the younger age group. They need friends badly, because the widow is often a social misfit who does not get invited out. This social isolation should be broken, especially at Christmas, and in the case of young widows, with baby-sitting help. Only 6% of women who are widowed between twenty and fifty years of age will eventually remarry. They are a potentially very lonely group. If grief is further complicated by financial hardship due to the death of the breadwinner, considerable support will be needed from social workers, health visitors, child guidance officers, housing departments and many others.[338]

Another organization, which helps the parents of dead or chronically ill children, is the Society of Compassionate Friends,† founded in 1969 by the Rev. Simon Stephens. Cruse is a service of counselling by professionals, whereas the Compassionate Friends is a self-help organization for parents. Such magnificent institutions as these are long overdue, and more help is still needed for the older age

* Head Office: Cruse House, 126 Sheen Road, Richmond, Surrey (01-940 4818).
† Head Office: 50 Woodwaye, Watford, Hertfordshire WD1 4NW. Phone: Watford (92 in London, 0923 on STD) 24279.

groups of widows and widowers. They help people over some of the most painful experiences of life. For bereavement can feel like mutilation. Similar patterns of grieving are indeed experienced by people who have lost a limb or a home.[281] The person's whole balance of health is disturbed. During the first six months of bereavement the death rate among widowers in one study was 40% higher than expected. They died mainly from coronary thromboses – broken hearts in every sense.[58] Widows have more trouble from their arthritis, asthma and ulcerative colitis than do their married counterparts,[219] requiring double the number of medical consultations for their osteoarthritis.[83] It has even been suggested that grief can occasionally cause or precipitate cancer, especially in people with personalities which do not respond aggressively to stress.[213]

A wide variety of psychiatric illnesses may also be precipitated by a bereavement, though it is possible that the person had them in a mild form before the stress of grief was added.[277] Dr George Engel found that actual pain may be experienced, sometimes mimicking that of the deceased person.[108]

One particularly difficult day is the first anniversary of the death. A visit from a friend, clergyman or doctor is then welcomed, and some hospices send a postcard with an offer of help if needed. The first Christmas can also be a barren time. Friends should offer hospitality and dinner on Christmas Day, but not take offence if it is rejected.

After a year or so, it may eventually be appropriate to point out to a person who is still grieving that their duty to the dead is now done and grieving has gone on long enough. A memorial service or a visit to the grave may help with making the break. It is now time to turn out to other people again; to redecorate the house.

Pathological Grief

The bereaved searches the time before the death for evidence of failure to do right by the lost one. He accuses himself of negligence and exaggerates minor omissions. After the fire disaster the central topic of discussion for a young married woman was the fact that her husband died after he left her following a quarrel, and of a young man whose wife died that he fainted too soon to save her.

By appropriate techniques these distorted pictures can be successfully transformed into a normal grief reaction with resolution. – Dr Erich Lindemann[219]

This transformation is effected mainly by someone who is prepared to listen without criticism to the bitterness and guilt which the bereaved person pours out. He finds that it is safe to let out these bottled-up feelings and is free to get on with his 'grief work'.

If it proceeds normally and is fully resolved, grief should be a healing response. But there are factors which can distort it, prolong it, or make it lead to physical and psychiatric disease.[121] Quite the most fascinating example in history is Queen Victoria, who remained depressed and in widow's black for forty years.

When the death is violent or preceded by disfigurement, this aspect may haunt a survivor and need to be talked about.[286]

Grieving people are more likely to need the help of a psychiatrist than they were before the bereavement.[277] Women, particularly younger ones, are thought to be more prone to this than men, at least in the first year. A number of situations may alert one to a danger of psychiatric disturbance with abnormally long or intense grieving.[287] For instance, if there is obvious animosity between the dying person and the survivor, then the latter is apt to suffer afterwards from feelings of anger or guilt. People who have very intense pining or who have grief-prone personalities that have reacted badly to loss in the past especially need to be befriended. So do those who are socially isolated or in whom the phase of depression leads to a withdrawn or 'living in the past' attitude. They, and people who feel guilty for stopping their mourning, are liable to sink into a state of perpetual grief which robs them of joy for life. This is a particular risk with the elderly, and might possibly be averted by regular visits from a health visitor who could also ensure that they eat an adequate diet.[11]

The normal process of unlearning the urge to recover the dead person can be impeded if an abnormal stimulus to the memory is encountered, leading to chronic grief. For this reason widows should be discouraged from attending spiritualist seances and the like. Even if some part of the dead man's personality is being contacted, it cannot be a part of any importance, since the 'messages' passed on are such inconsequential rubbish.

There is a current vogue, perhaps because of the failure of the Churches to speak to the condition of most modern people, for dabbling in this 'spooky' side of death. Particularly in America at present there is a danger that instead of receiving help for their self-evident needs, the dying and bereaved may be led into a world of fantasy and pseudo-religion. Spirit presences, silver cords, beings of light, out-of-the-body experiences and communication with the dead have stimulated a great library of journalism and even some research, regrettably backed by a few august scientists whose erudition and experience is beyond reproach. I do not dismiss what they have found as untrue – all these things may well exist – but as irrelevant. I do not, by my deathbed, want someone ecstatic about life *after* death, but someone who will pull their finger out and ensure that I do not suffer before it. Not without reason have the great religions discouraged men from dabbling in necromancy (e.g. Deut. 18–11) because there are few more potent dreams for turning attention away from our duties in this life. 'The ignorant man,' says the Katha Upanishad, 'runs after pleasure, sinks into the entanglements of death; but the wise man, seeking the undying, does not run among things that die.'* When a man dies, he has departed. He only leaves behind the things that die, be it a putrefying corpse or the wrinkles in the substance of mind which distinguished his personality. To go on troubling whatever remains of him in the world of mind is as indecent as sleeping with his corpse. The experiences people are describing in this field, while no doubt true, are being wrongly interpreted to them. We lack the wise men to do this interpreting. Meanwhile the whole process, though perhaps comforting some, may well protract and render unhealthy the grieving of many.

Dickens furnished us with a splendid description of chronic grief in *The Old Curiosity Shop*, though it is often more painful than this:

... she told her how she had wept and moaned and prayed to die herself, when this had happened; and how when she first came to that place (the graveside of her husband), a young creature strong in love and grief, she had hoped that her heart was breaking as it seemed to be. But that time passed by, and although she continued to be sad when she came there, still she could bear to come, and so went on until it was pain no longer, but a solemn pleasure, and a duty she had learned to like. And now that five-and-fifty years were gone, she spoke of the dead man as if he had been her son or grandson, with a kind of pity for his youth ...

In this state a widow may be hallucinated with visions of the dead, though simple illusions of his presence are more common. She conceives her duty to be towards the man who has gone rather than towards the all-too-pressing needs of those still living.

Another kind of bereavement which often causes trouble is the death of a child.[16] 'Cot deaths', accidents or teenage suicides are particularly traumatic for the parents, who may feel guilty and desperate, sometimes even committing suicide themselves. 'Why was I not more careful or more understanding?' they ask. If no one listens to this

*W. B. Yeats, *The Ten Principal Upanishads*, Faber, 1937, p. 33.

tirade of self-reproach, it may become a lifelong burden. If the marriage is already under strain, or if the dead child was an only child, the problem is even worse.[263]

The child found dead in his cot for no apparent reason is causing concern to modern paediatricians. To the distress of the family are added the humiliating implications of a coroner's investigation. When he decides it was a 'cot death' the coroner will frequently refer the family to a paediatrician interested in the problem, who can reassure them and compare their case with other similar ones.[47] An organization has been founded in London to deal with these emergencies.* It has research and welfare departments.

Grieving Children

Grief in children is more likely to follow pathological patterns.[32] There is some evidence that infants in particular tend to suppress grief, so that it manifests much later as an apparently unrelated symptom.[29] The same reactions can be sparked off by temporary separation from the mother, observation of which has led to the present-day concern over 'maternal deprivation'.[38] The same problems can arise, however, in children separated from other familiar elements in their environment, and the whole topic is being currently reconsidered. The result, however, may perhaps be psychiatric or even criminal behaviour in later life.[53] It was found, for instance, that one third of the women in Holloway Prison were fatherless. If it is the father who dies, someone in the child's life may be needed to fill some of his functions, even if only seen infrequently. A psychiatrist, family doctor or priest may be able to be the source of advice, direction and discipline which is needed. One organization which comes near to replacing the father is the Australian institution 'Legacy', which enabled servicemen who had survived the war to

* Foundation for the Study of Infant Deaths, 23 St Peter's Square, London W6 9NW (01-235 1721).

give long-term support to the widows and children of their comrades who had died. Small children often appear to 'get over' a bereavement more quickly than an adult, and certainly should not have a duty to grieve imposed on them by adults. If they are playing happily, this is good. They soon re-attach themselves to a substitute for the dead person. When it is someone really vital, like a mother, who has died, what is needed is a new, reliable and unchanging mother figure as soon as possible.

An even more common problem is that of the child who is excluded from any family grieving because adults feel, quite wrongly, that they should not cry in front of him. He can feel very shut out. So children do need permission to grieve, but they should not be expected to grieve on an adult pattern because they may not be all that much upset.

It is commonly supposed that if the death is hushed up and never mentioned, the child will not grieve, but this could not be further from the truth.[405] It may be noted that his school performance deteriorates, and that he manifests anxiety. Children aged between six and ten are apt to feel guilty about the death, and to wonder whether it was something that they did which caused it – an anxiety which can be easily relieved if detected. It is essential to be frank with children, and to let them grieve with the parents, who need not be afraid to show distress or to talk about their sorrow.

In terms of subsequent mental health, the death of a parent is more damaging to the children than is divorce.[102] At least the departure of one parent in a divorce brings relief from bickering and is accompanied by a sense of 'Thank heaven he's gone.' But in the case of a death, there is the grief of the surviving parent to cope with. At first because of depression and disorganization, and later because of the added burden of being both mother and father – both housekeeper and breadwinner – the surviving parent will have less time for the children. They can easily feel starved of affection. If it was another child that died, the surviving brothers and sisters may feel insecure – perhaps they might die too? – and are often more clinging and conscious of their own health, making parents irritable. If the parents are also carrying a burden of guilt because they treated the initial symptoms of the dead child's illness as behaviour problems, they may experience serious inner conflict.

So how can one help a bereaved child? First and foremost by helping the parent.[33] In, for example, a Cruse Parents' Circle, a widow can receive practical and emotional help. She may perhaps speak out about her angry and even murderous feelings towards the surviving children when they are being difficult. Then, feeling understood herself, she can go home and be more affectionate to the children. What must be established is free communication about their grief between parents and children: a two-way listening. It helps to express grief, to talk about the dead person, to cry together.

Sometimes it helps for an outside counsellor to speak to the child on his own,[34] but most of the support will usually grow between the family members themselves. If they do not do this from the start, great tensions may arise as no one considers anyone else. If the child entertains fantasies that the death was in some way caused by something he did, it is nearly always easy to put right the misunderstanding. One can say that the dead person did not want to die, and that his death is not anyone's fault, but the most important rule is to let the child talk about it. Find out what he thinks about it, either in conversing with him, or in watching what ideas he expresses in games where death is included. Playing games about people dying is one way children come to terms with the idea; they should not be discouraged. It is exceptional for a child to be feeling guilt about a death, but when he does express it, reassurance is usually readily accepted.

One bereavement is enough. Moving house, putting the child into care, breaking up the family, can all put a strain on the child by forcing him into even bigger adjustments. It is a good general rule to avoid any drastic changes for at least six months. Remember also that, as with adults, grief may continue for much longer than that.

Helping the Grief of the Dying

As I pointed out in Chapter 4 (pp. 58–9), the dying man will be grieving as surely as his relatives. This will be hardest for the person who is leaving a successful, well integrated life with strong ties to people and possessions. As Dr C. Knight Aldrich wrote: 'Strength of personality may help a patient not so much to avoid depression in anticipation of death as to conceal the depression from others.'[6] Perhaps the way to help in making this grief bearable is to enable the dying man to feel useful to other people. I have known many dying patients who taught students on ward rounds with great zest, telling them about pain control, why they no longer believed in euthanasia, and how they were being helped to face death themselves.

A dying person can help his family to begin to anticipate what life will be like without him. If he has discussed with his wife her plans for the future and the provisions in his will, it will be much easier for her to adjust to her future as a widow. Just before he died, Hans Zinsser, an American bacteriologist, consoled his wife by writing sonnets for her. Here are some of his lines: [436]

> When I am gone – and I shall go before you –
> Think of me not as your disconsolate lover;
> Think of the joy it gave me to adore you,
> Of sun and stars you helped me to discover.
>
> And this still living part of me will come
> To sit beside you, in the empty room.
>
> Then all on Earth that Death has left behind
> Will be the merry part of me within your mind.

The Need for Mourning

Traditional patterns of living usually incorporate a means of formal expression of grief. There was the Victorian funeral, with its hearse and flowers and black crape; the prescribed oration of the Kaddish in the Orthodox Synagogue service, to be spoken by a recently-bereaved Jew every week for eleven months and on the anniversary of the death; the pomp and dignity of state funerals; the old Irish keening wake in which women swayed all night in a trance-like state, chanting dirges.

Every culture has had its equivalent ceremony, but today in Britain this need is frequently unsatisfied. The bereaved are avoided, with their grief bottled up, like a poison which, instead of being thrown out by the body, stays to damage it.[136] Somehow we manage to ignore death. We rarely see anyone die; most of us have never seen a corpse; we seldom teach our medical students anything about it.[350, 415] In American funeral parlours cosmetics and smile-fixers are used on the corpse to reinforce this great denial.[258]

Our lack of such ceremonies means that some people need help to get past these difficult milestones in life.

One of the doctor's principal functions in atypical or unresolved grief reactions is to catalyze the normal expression of sorrow. If he is to do this effectively, the physician will need to have a positive inclination to foster the emotional expression of sorrow. He needs to have much the same enthusiasm for incising and draining a well-encapsulated pocket of grief as for incising a ripe and accessible abscess.[229]

The bereaved Jew and his family have clearly defined duties throughout the period of mourning, and each knows what is expected of him. In Victorian England the rituals of mourning were even more rigid, as these passages from Spon's *Household Manual* of 1894 show:

A widow's mourning is the deepest, and continued longest. For the first twelve months the dress and the mantle must be of paramatta, the skirt of the dress covered with crape, put on in one piece to within an inch of the waist; sleeves tight to the arm, bodice entirely covered with crape ... and deep lawn collar. The mantle ... is very heavily trimmed with crape. The widow's cap must be worn for a year, but not beyond the year. At the end of the sixth month (eighteen months in all) crape may be left off, and plain black worn for six months: and two years complete the period of mourning. For the first year, while a widow wears her weeds, she can, of course, accept no invitations; and it is in the worst possible taste for her to be seen in any place of public resort. After the first year she can, if so disposed, gradually resume her place in society.[357]

Even the width of the black edging round the mourner's visiting card, and the depth of mourning appropriate for a second cousin were laid down meticulously. Grief was made external to the person, formalized and thus 'detoxicated'. Nowadays we often do not even say farewells.

To counter this trend, hospices nearly all have a 'viewing chapel' where the body, not degraded by cosmetics or other attempts to conceal what it is, is decently laid out so that family members may, if they wish, take their leave. Many undertakers have 'chapels of rest' for the same purpose. Prayers can be repeated, if required, in privacy.

While nobody who wishes to see the dead body of a loved person should be denied, not every relative will wish to do so and all concerned should be sensitive to individual feelings in the matter. Some may prefer to remember him as he was rather than as his body appeared after he was gone. Children are especially vulnerable. If someone can say, 'he's gone and his body is all peaceful now', they will also be able to see whether the bereaved child needs proof of that statement. Most are helped by saying a formal goodbye.

The English like to grieve in staunch silence, but this is not a universal behaviour pattern, and people should be allowed to grieve in their own way. I can remember a horrified nun in St Joseph's Hospice who recounted how seventeen members of an old Italian grandfather's family gradually gathered round his bed during his last night. They waited tense and poised as his breathing failed. Sister knelt beside him, repeated the prayers for the dying and felt his pulse. It flickered to a stop and she said, 'He's gone now', whereupon the entire company burst out howling and two disconsolate women hurled themselves whooping across his chest in paroxysms of remorse. The corpse took a mighty gasping breath and uttered a final satisfied groan.

> Beyond the shadows of this world,
> Within our reach, a radiance shines.
> Could we but lift the veil and see,
> And know that shade with light combines
> To make us whole. It must be so.
> In dark skies, only, stars will glow.

Ethel Waddington Lamerton, *Light and Darkness*[200]

12. The Place of Religion

❈

All beings are invisible before their birth and after death are invisible again. They are seen between two unseens. Why in this find cause for grief? ... The Spirit that is in all creatures is immortal in them all. Why grieve for the death of that which cannot die? – *Bhagavad Gita*, Chapter 2

The greatest pain of all, which I mentioned in Chapter 4, comes from a great inner longing. This feeling of lack, or inadequacy, or sin, or however it expresses itself, can best be ministered to from one of the great religious teachings. We have built ourselves a fortress of personality in which to hide and have thought of ourselves as only a body which we feed, pamper, adorn and display with all our energy. When the body is spoiled and the fortress crumbles, we are compelled to search for something more permanent than either. For many of us the shackles of complacency will never be shaken by anything short of death, but at that point even the toughest old sinner may have a question or two. Mr R., the old Glaswegian convict whose story I told earlier, said to me one day, after a little reflection, 'Recently I've thought about religion, because I'm nearing death.'

Which Religion?

There are many practical points in the care of patients who are adherents of different faiths.

Roman Catholics have merged Extreme Unction with the Anointing of the Sick which can if appropriate lead into Communion, Confession and Absolution. This wise arrangement will give great comfort to the relatives, without unduly frightening the patient. It is desirable that a priest be present with a dying Catholic. If none is available then anyone may encourage the patient to ask forgiveness for sins. And incidentally, cremation is permissible for Catholics nowadays. The Anglican approach is broadly similar, but is less likely to be so formalized unless the patient requests the sacraments. Having no ritual framework, the Nonconformist minister is thrown back on his own wisdom, resource and goodness. All may use the reading of scripture.[270]

> And I heard a great voice out of heaven saying,
> Behold, the tabernacle of God is with men, and he
> will dwell with them, and they shall be his people,
> and God himself shall be with them, and be their God.
>
> And God shall wipe away all tears from their eyes;
> and there shall be no more death, neither sorrow, nor
> crying, neither shall there be any more pain: for the
> former things are passed away.
>
> Revelation 21 : 3–4

Rabbis will also wish to read a confessional service, acknowledging the need for spiritual healing. In the case of an Orthodox Jew, the body may be removed to the mortuary, with the arms and hands extended at the sides of the body,[269] but cleansing will be carried out by members of a special Burial Society. Dissection or removal of any organs except the cornea is avoided. Preferably the body should not be left unattended until the funeral. Burial follows, and should be as soon as possible. Liberal Jews relax most of these rules. After the death will come the period of Shiva described on page 185.

> The Lord gave, and the Lord hath taken away;
> blessed be the Name of the Lord.
>
> Job 1 : 21

Moslems have even stricter rules: [2, 21] the Imam will usually tell the patient that he will soon die, and urge him to confess sins and beg forgiveness. If at all possible, the family should be present when he dies, and thereafter they must wash and prepare the body. It will be left facing Mecca and only relatives or friends should move it. No infidel should touch the body, but usually families are at a loss and only too glad to be shown what to do. 'Facing Mecca' in Britain means that the feet will be pointing to the south east and the head raised on one pillow. A post mortem must be avoided at all costs; not even the cornea may be removed. Moslems are always buried rather than cremated, usually with no coffin.

> Believers, fear Allah and trust his Apostle.
> He will grant you a double measure of his
> mercy; He will guide your steps with light,
> and will forgive you: Allah is the Compassionate,
> the Merciful.

Koran, Chapter 57

In order to enter his next life in a good state, the Buddhist needs, above all, to die happy. When the patient is found to have a terminal illness, a Buddhist monk from the nearest Vihara should be asked to befriend him. At the appropriate time he will want to recite Sutras and bless the patient, asking him to recall his *good* deeds. A monk with a picture of the Buddha will try to be present at the moment of death, but afterwards all funeral services are considered as grief therapy for the relatives. Autopsies are permitted.

> If you rest in the stillness like a broken gong, you have
> already reached heaven, for anger has left you. Like a
> cowherd, driving his cows to the pastures, old age and death
> drive men to new life.

Dhammapada, vv. 134–5

Hindus have a more exacting ritual. The Guru may tie a thread round the neck or wrist of the patient to signify a blessing. The thread should not be removed. Immediately after death he will pour water into the mouth of the body, while the family wash it. As many Hindus are particular about who should touch the body, one should ask first. They will require a cremation as soon as possible.

It was not born; it will never die; once having been it can never cease to be. Beginningless, unchanging, endless, yet most ancient, the Spirit does not die when the body is dead. – *Bhagavad Gita*, Chapter 2

While the various observances of different religions are almost quaint in their differences, it is what they have in common that is most impressive. All religions demand that those ministering to the dying shall preserve as peaceful an atmosphere as possible for the patient. Afterwards, they all agree that the body must be treated with respect and gentleness. The reason for this latter is generally forgotten, but a Moslem will insist that although the connection between mind and body is broken at death, the actual separation takes much longer, and any carelessness in handling the corpse is felt as keenly by the patient as if he were alive.

Further, all the religions require that a dying man should go humbly, even apologetically, regretting folly but at the same time confident and rejoicing in divine Mercy. A man *in extremis* knows that he cannot get away with anything, that God is not mocked. If he knows about Justice (and in Britain everyone does) he may reasonably be terrified. The only consolation he could possibly be given in the light of this knowledge is to be reminded that Justice is only an aspect of Mercy, that this is the first quality radiated by the Godhead, and that it is boundless, without measure.

However, while this is fine for those who have a formalized faith, most of us are only vaguely Christian. To such, religion can be a help, perhaps proving at last a gateway to the inner treasure house. For such people religion must always be available, but never force-fed.

Daily prayers in terminal wards are universally appreciated. Though some people do not take part, I have never
heard anyone object. When a 'nominal C. of E.' patient
dies, an obvious need can be filled by familiar, non-
sectarian prayers, and the joyful comfort of the twenty-
third psalm. The chaplain (or the local vicar[127] if the
patient is at home) should therefore introduce himself at
least socially to every patient.

To our surprise, as we cared for patients dying at home
in East London in 1978, we found ourselves cooperating
with a clergyman in some 31% of cases, the corresponding
figure for 1977 being 25%. Considering that only 8% of
the population in the area are churchgoers, this indicates
a remarkably efficient grapevine. The clergy are to be
complimented on the sensitivity of their antennae.

The Natural Religion

The chaplain of one hospice said that people who had not
given a thought to religion, and those with a very strong
religion, died more peacefully than those with a luke-
warm faith whose ill-considered assumptions collapsed
under stress. This observation was confirmed statistically
by Professor Hinton.[158] But the most interesting group,
the chaplain continued, were the three or four firm
atheists whom he had seen die. Without exception they
became enraged, and died in turmoil.

Because of his special training, a clergyman is a valuable member of the team. Without him we would find our
job much harder. He will try to show the patient that
'While I thought I was learning how to live, I was learning how to die,' as Leonardo da Vinci expressed it. He will
help him 'to eliminate from his life – his actual present
earthly life – all the elements of destruction, and of decay,
corruption, bitterness, resentment and hatred: all those
things which kill a soul'.[36] Of course if no priest is available, or if the patient cannot accept one, there is no reason
why other members of the caring team should not give

this help. The message may be, 'I don't know why this is happening; but I know it will be *all right*.'[112]

All that I have said in previous chapters about counselling – of both the dying and the bereaved – could be the function of the clergyman, who is often the member of the team most suited to the task. It is a matter of uncovering hidden inner knowledge.

In the depth of your hopes and desires lies your silent knowledge of the beyond; And like seeds dreaming beneath the snow your heart dreams of spring. Trust the dreams, for in them is hidden the gate to eternity.

Your fear of death is but the trembling of the shepherd when he stands before the king whose hand is to be laid upon him in honour. Is the shepherd not joyful beneath his trembling, that he shall wear the mark of the king? Yet is he not more mindful of his trembling?

For what is it to die but to stand naked in the wind and to melt into the sun? And what is it to cease breathing but to free the breath from its restless tides, that it may rise and expand and seek God unencumbered?

Kahlil Gibran, *The Prophet*

So much for people with a formal religion. But we are now seeing increasing numbers of people who can believe in nothing but the body and personality. For a Christian to try to communicate in these circumstances can be like trying to talk to an uncomprehending foreigner. It can be disconcerting when all one's beliefs and terminology are questioned.

The Romans met this problem when they established law courts in new colonies. Some of the disputes arising knew no precedent in Roman Law. So they fell back on the traditional laws of the colonists, the Jus Gentium. But if there was no guide there either, the judge would appeal to Jus Naturale: the natural justice self-evident to all men.

There is a parallel here. If a man has a religion, we must respect and obey it. But if he has none, we have to fall back on the Natural Religion, because his needs are still the same. That is to say that you have to answer the patient's questions, or face his fears, quite naked of comfortably formalized ideas. You have to speak the Truth as you know it at the time, fresh and alive; precisely appropriate to this man and his present needs.

13. What is Death?

In a little while I will be gone from you, my people, and whither I cannot tell. From nowhere we come; into nowhere we go. What is life? It is the flash of a firefly in the night. It is the breath of the buffalo in the winter-time. It is the shadow that runs across the grass and loses itself in the sunset. – Chief Crowfoot

If we would care for the dying we must first bring order to our own philosophy about death.[113] Caring for a man in trouble means facing trouble with him. If we cannot face it, we will fail him. But having a philosophy does not mean having all the answers. It means holding to principles, and being content to fill in the details later should they ever be needed.

What Happens?

The only natural cause of death is old age, but it is uncommon to die of this, and to judge by his statistical reports, the Registrar General doesn't believe in it at all! (See p. 133, Figure C.) Most of us die of disease of some kind, unless we meet death suddenly in an accident. When the death is not sudden, it is evident that it proceeds in distinct stages. Even physical death advances by degrees. Organs fail at different rates, and when the body begins to die it does so from below upwards. Use of the legs is lost before that of the arms, the abdominal organs cease to function before those in the chest, the feet are cold before the head.

A man's mind may be intact until the body dies, or it may disintegrate first, sometimes very gradually. The death of the personality can appear like death of the man himself if we have never looked at the person more deeply than to see his social machinery. Like the body, however, the personality is just a bag of tools. The blunting of these instruments has rarely been so well described as in a Personal Paper in the *Lancet* some years ago.[12]

This mind is not dependent on the body for its life. If the mind is disturbed enough, the body will die, as the practice of voodoo magic has shown. Harvey Cox wrote:

Anthropologists who investigate magical beliefs among tribal peoples today report that violating a taboo can cause death, and that people who have been killed in effigy by voodoo techniques do in fact die with more than accidental frequency. The reason for this is that a personality system includes organic, social and cultural components. A person whose whole view of himself includes the cultural meanings inherent in a magical society will literally die if that culture indicates he should. Culture has a powerful effect on persons, far more than we were willing to admit during the eighteenth and nineteenth centuries, when rationalistic individualism laughed at such things.[69]

A scientific look at people with a predilection to death has shown that such forces also operate in our own society, if more hidden.[5]

To tell us what happens at death, who better than someone who has encountered it. A friend of mine was drowned, but resuscitated, so I asked him to write down what he experienced. Here is his account:

When I was seven years old, I used to go to a boating pond in the local park; for six pennies I could take out a boat for half an hour.

On one occasion, my boat got stuck at the side of the bank, and in attempting to push myself free, I overturned the boat and fell into the water. The water was not very deep, but I was fully submerged until I was pulled free by somebody, probably the park-keeper. I do not know how long I stayed below the surface of the pond, it could have been less than a minute. However, I shall describe the episode *as I experienced it,* and not as it 'must' or 'should' have been.

I recall an element of surprise, but not panic or fear. Nor did I feel any physical pain or suffering of any kind. Nevertheless, I had a sense that death was near. At some point I became aware of my whole body as being separate from me, and this awareness extended to include children playing in a nearby shallow pond. I was aware of trees surrounding the pond, the covering sky, groups of people and a woman walking along pushing a pram. This awareness was extended as much underwater as above it: in particular, a small fish swam into view. I became acutely conscious that the feeling of my own being included that of this creature; in fact, there were not two separate beings, only one, although the *body* of the fish and *my* body were separate. This *knowledge* communicated itself *mutually,* as a felt experience.

Throughout this period, I was making no effort to save myself. I felt embraced by a Great Presence in which I experienced utter peace; a pure, still joy to which the normal experiences of pleasure or happiness bear no relation, and yet I cannot remember anything so thrilling; and the certainty of absolute invulnerability – nothing, but nothing, could as much as scratch what I am. This Presence was, although possessing no form, *not* impersonal: the inclination is to say He, rather than It. I was fully known by this Presence which had enveloped me with such love and care.

Whilst in this state, I experienced visually my entire childhood; imagine a film of seven years' duration seen in the 'twinkling of an eye'! Yet it was more than visual, for I was left with a 'taste', a kind of distilled quality or essence of those years. This was just observed – I do not recall any value-judgement about it.

On a few occasions since this experience, I have known that sense of complete invulnerability, already referred to. It has arisen in moments of actual or possible danger.

Death is a Mystery

To die is different from what anyone supposed – and luckier.
– Walt Whitman

By the Law of England a man is dead when two doctors, with no professional or other interest in his death, have pronounced him dead. The Bar Council has firmly declined to define death more precisely than that, and as far as I know, no one else has ever done better. (Recent experience in intensive care units, for instance, has shown that the electro-encephalogram is at best only an indicator, with no absolute authority.)[182] The fact that such difficulty is encountered in defining death suggests that we are dealing with something mysterious. The modern mind dislikes mysteries. Even our architecture banishes dark corners: everything has to be flat and open. But death *is* a mystery.

On one of the few occasions when I heard a patient ask 'Am I dying?' the doctor's reply was 'No. But your body soon will.' In this form, the message was acceptable, and did not give rise to despair or fear. Only when we give the name 'I' to something which is not 'I' can death be fearful.

Birth forces the baby out of the protective seclusion of the womb into the human family: death forces the same individual out of a now familiar society into the unknown, leaving behind a physical body to disintegrate in a tomb and some sort of a gap in that society, which others in their turn will fill ... It is entirely natural and understandable that we should feel afraid of death, for it mutilates body and mind, which together form our image of ourselves as 'us', it forces us to leave those near and dear to us and the familiar world around us, and to give up our hold on life as we know it.[405]

An eddy in a turbulent river has its own sound and its own form, and its special relationship with other swirling eddies, then it rejoins the great river. Perhaps it grieves! The traditional answer to such mysteries – that when you die you go to heaven, as John Smith, recognizable and still separate, possibly with a purgatorial wait first – does not satisfy many people nowadays. Where such simple faith survives it is beautiful, appropriate and deeply to be respected, but the idea no longer rings true to most people.[112]

This is no cause for sadness, since the idea was at best an attempt to express the inexpressible. It never could be more than an allegory. We should therefore look to see what truth it was trying to portray, and how this can be reinterpreted to people of today.

So, What is Death?

If humanism were right in declaring that man is born to be happy, he would not be born to die. Since his body is doomed to die, his task on earth evidently must be of a more spiritual nature. It cannot be unrestrained enjoyment of everyday life. It cannot be the search for the best ways to obtain material goods and then cheerfully get the most out of them. It has to be the fulfilment of a permanent, earnest duty so that one's life journey may become an experience of moral growth, so that one may leave life a better human being than one started it. – Alexander Solzhenitsyn

To care for the dying is a very human occupation which offers an opportunity for pure giving, because the dying man can never repay what he receives.

At the hour of our death the great need is for stillness, and that is available in abundance. *Peace I leave with you, my peace I give unto you: not as the world giveth give I unto you. Let not your heart be troubled, neither let it be afraid.* – John 14.27.

In the moment of death, something departs, leaving the body behind. It is the moment when a man leaves his body. Death is therefore a change of form. It is widely believed that a soul survives, in some other form. In the East it has always been held that the soul returns to manifest again in a new body.

Plato also deduced this, as he recounted in Book Ten of *The Republic* – the daughter of Necessity is speaking to the dead:

Souls of a day, a new generation of men shall here begin the cycle of its mortal existence. Your destiny shall not be allotted to you: you shall choose it freely for yourselves. Let him who draws the first lot be the first to choose his next life which shall be his irrevocably. But virtue owns no master: as a man honours or slights her, so he shall have more of her or less. The responsibility lies with the chooser: Heaven is blameless ... it was a truly amazing sight to watch how each soul selected its life – a sight at once sad, and ludicrous, and strange, for the choice was largely governed by the habits of their previous life.

Plato's scheme certainly has its appeal, since it displays absolute Justice, yet permits of unimpeded improvement by postulating a dimension beyond time.

Whatever one believes, all great teachers have accepted that the dying man must prepare for another world. Never should this preparation be interfered with. It is helped by simple qualities such as goodness and beauty, with which we should surround the dying. The traditional symbols and ceremonies of our religions provide for this need. At death a man's mental possessions all fall away, so that when he really is dying he should be given only the Truth, not what we suppose might please him – there is nothing left which can be pleased or displeased.

And I repeat, he needs us to be still.

So: What is Death?

Bibliography

ANTHONY, S., *The Discovery of Death in Childhood and After*, Penguin Education, London, 1973.

AUTTON, NORMAN, *The Pastoral Care of the Dying*, SPCK, London, 1966.

AUTTON, NORMAN, *The Pastoral Care of the Bereaved*, SPCK, London, 1967.

*BURTON, LINDY, *Care of the Child Facing Death*, Routledge & Kegan Paul, London, 1974.

CAINE, LYNN, *Widow*, William Mower, New York, 1974.

CANCER CARE INC. (1 Park Avenue, New York 10016), *Catastrophic Illness in the Seventies – Symposium*, 1971.

*CARTWRIGHT, A., et al., *Life Before Death*, Routledge & Kegan Paul, London, 1973.

CHURCH INFORMATION OFFICE (Church House, Dean's Yard, London SW1), *On Dying Well*.

*COLLIN, RODNEY, *The Theory of Eternal Life*, Stuart & Watkins, London, 1956.

CONSUMERS ASSOCIATION (14 Buckingham Street, London WC2), *What to Do When Someone Dies*.

DE BEAUVOIR, S., *A Very Easy Death*, Warner Books, New York, 1973.

D.H.S.S., *Care of the Dying – Proceedings of a National Symposium*, 29 November 1972, H.M. Stationery Office, London.

DOWNIE, P. A., *Cancer Rehabilitation*, Faber & Faber, London, 1978.

DOWNING, A. B. (ed.), *Euthanasia and the Right to Death*, Peter Owen, London, 1969.

FORD, ARTHUR, *The Life Beyond Death*, Berkley, New York, 1971.

GIBRAN, KAHLIL, *The Prophet*, Heinemann, London, 1926.

HINTON, JOHN, *Dying*, Penguin, London, 1967.

KELLY, ORVILLE E., *Make Today Count*, Delacorte Press, New York, 1975.

*KÜBLER-ROSS, ELISABETH, *On Death and Dying*, Tavistock Publications, London, 1970.

*KÜBLER-ROSS, ELISABETH, *Questions and Answers on Death and Dying*, Macmillan, London, 1974.

KÜBLER-ROSS, ELISABETH (ed.), *Death: The Final Stage of Growth*, Prentice-Hall International, Spectrum Books, London, 1975.

LACK, SYLVIA, & BUCKINGHAM, ROBERT, *First American Hospice*. From Hospice of Connecticut, 765 Prospect Street, New Haven, Connecticut 06511 (send $16).

LACK, S. A., & LAMERTON, R. C., *The Hour of Our Death*, Geoffrey Chapman, 1974. From St Joseph's Hospice, Mare Street, London E8.

LANGONE, J., *Death is a Noun*, Dell, New York, 1972.

LEWIS, C. S., *The Problem of Pain*, Fontana, London, 1940.

LEWIS, C. S., *A Grief Observed*, Faber & Faber, London, 1961.

MARRIS, P., *Widows and Their Families*, Routledge, London, 1958.

MARTINSON, I. M. (ed.), *Home Care for the Dying Child*, Appleton-Century-Crofts, New York, 1976.

MITFORD, JESSICA, *The American Way of Death*, Fawcett, Greenwich, Connecticut, 1963.

NIGHTINGALE, FLORENCE, *Notes on Nursing*, Blackie, London, 1974.

MOODY, RAYMOND A., *Life After Life*, Corgi, London, 1976.

MOODY, RAYMOND A., *Reflections on Life After Life*, Corgi, London, 1978.

*PARKES, COLIN M., *Bereavement*, Tavistock Publications, London, 1972.

*PINCUS, LILY, *Death and the Family*, Random House, Pantheon Books, New York, 1974.

ROSEN, R. D., *Psychobabble*, Atheneum, New York, 1977.

RUSSELL, O. R., *Freedom to Die*, Human Sciences Press, New York, 1977.

ST. JOHN-STEVAS, NORMAN, *The Right to Life*, Hodder, London, 1963.

SAUNDERS, CICELY, *Care of the Dying*, Nursing Times Booklet, 1976.

**SAUNDERS, CICELY (ed.), *The Management of Terminal Disease*, Edward Arnold, London, 1978.

*SOLZHENITSYN, A., *Cancer Ward*, Bodley Head, London, 1968.

SPECK, PETER, *Loss and Grief in Medicine*, Baillière Tindall, London, 1978.

*STEPHENS, SIMON, *Death Comes Home*, Mowbrays, London, 1972.

*STODDARD, SANDOL, *The Hospice Movement*, Jonathan Cape, London, 1979.

*TORRIE, MARGARET, *Begin Again*, Dent, London, 1970.

TROWELL, HUGH, *The Unfinished Debate on Euthanasia*, 1973, SCM Press, 56 Bloomsbury Street, London WC1.

TWYCROSS, ROBERT G., *The Dying Patient*, Christian Medical Fellowship Booklet, 157 Waterloo Road, London SE1.

VERE, D. W. (ed.), *Topics in Therapeutics*, 4, Pitman Medical Booklet, P.O. Box 7, Tunbridge Wells, Kent, England.

WAMBACH, HELEN, *Life Before Life*, Bantam, London, 1979.

WERTHAM, F., *The German Euthanasia Program*, Hayes, 6304 Hamilton Avenue, Cincinnati, Ohio 45224, 1978.

WILLIAMS, GLANVILLE, *The Sanctity of Life and the Criminal Law*, Faber & Faber, London, 1958.

*WORCESTER, ALFRED, *The Care of the Aged, the Dying and the Dead*, Blackwell Scientific Publications, Oxford, 1935.

References

Volume numbers of journals are in bold type. The following abbreviations have been used:

C.M.A.J.   Canadian Medical Association Journal
P.R.S.M.   Proceedings of the Royal Society of Medicine
J.M.E.   Journal of Medical Ethics
B.M.J.   British Medical Journal
J.(R.)C.G.P.   Journal of the (Royal) College of General Practitioners
N.M.   Nursing Mirror
N.T.   Nursing Times
J.A.M.A.   Journal of the American Medical Association
W.M.   World Medicine
A.J.N.   American Journal of Nursing

I have used references because they express a point of view better than I can, because they contain the results of the research upon which I base my statement, or because they expand more fully on a subject I could only mention briefly. Particularly valuable sources are marked with an asterisk. Two asterisks indicate a crucial work which helped to give direction to the whole field of care of the dying or the bereaved.

1. ADAMS, G. F., 'Personal View', *B.M.J.*, 1969, **4**, p. 363.
2. AHMED, K. S., 'Taking Medicines During Ramadan', *B.M.J.*, 1971, **4**, p. 425. (See also ref. 21.)
3. AITKEN-SWAN, J., *'Nursing the Late Cancer Patient at Home', *Practitioner*, 1959, **183**, p. 64. (See also refs. 56, 322.)
4. AITKEN-SWAN, J., and EASSON, E. C., *'Reactions of Cancer Patients on Being Told Their Diagnosis', *B.M.J.*, 1959, **1**, p. 779.
5. ALDERSON, M., 'Relationship Between Month of Birth and Month of Death in the Elderly', *British Journal of Preventive and Social Medicine*, 1975, **29**, p. 151. (See also refs. 49, 403.)
6. ALDRICH, C. K., *'The Dying Patient's Grief', *J.A.M.A.*, 1963, **184**, p. 329. (See also ref. 54.)
7. ALLEN, P., 'Too Many Elderly Patients to Care For?', *Modern Geriatrics*, 1976 (November), p. 15. (See also refs. 324, 411.)
8. ALSOFROM, J., 'The Hospice Way of Dying – At Home with Friends and Family', *American Medical News*, 1977, **20** (21 February), p. 7. (See also ref. 319.)
9. ALVAREZ, W. C., 'Care of the Dying', *J.A.M.A.*, 1952, **150**, p. 86.

10. AMULREE, Lord, 15th James Mackenzie Lecture, 16 November, 1968, *J.R.C.G.P.*, 1969, **17**, p. 3. (See also ref. 179.)

11. ANDERSON, W. F., 'A Death in the Family', *B.M.J.*, 1973, **1**, p. 31. (See also ref. 421.)

12. ANON, ******'Death of a Mind – Personal Paper', *Lancet*, 1950, **1**, p. 1012.

13. ANON, 'The Importance of Death', *W.M.*, 1968 (13 August), p. 24. (See also ref. 295.)

14. ANON, ******'Death In the First Person', *A.J.N.*, 1970, **70** (February), p. 336.

15. ARING, C. D., 'Intimations of Mortality', *Annals of Internal Medicine*, 1968, **69**, p. 137. (See also refs. 72, 205.)

16. ATKIN, M., 'The Doomed Family: Observations on the Lives of Parents and Children Facing Repeated Child Mortality'. Paper from 'Cruse', 126 Sheen Road, Richmond, Surrey, England. (See ref. 199.)

17. ATKIN, M., 'Counselling Families', *N.M.*, 1977 (7 April), p. 62.

18. BACON, F., 'Of Death', *Essaies of Sr. Francis Bacon*, John Beale, London, 1612. (See also ref. 258.)

19. BAILEY, M., *****'A Survey of the Social Needs of Patients with Incurable Lung Cancer', *Almoner*, 1959, **11**, p. 379.

20. BANKS, A.L., 'Euthanasia', *Practitioner*, 1948, **161**, p. 101.

21. BAQUI, A., 'Muslim Teaching Concerning Death', *N.T.*, 1979 (5 April), Occasional Papers Supplement.

22. BARCKLEY, V., 'Caring for the Cancer Patient At Home', *Journal of Practical Nursing*, 1974, **24** (October), p. 24.

23. BARNETT, S. W., *****'Euthanasia and the Last Weeks', letter to the *Guardian*, London, 1976 (22 November). (See also ref. 321.)

24. BARRETT, H., Second Annual Report of St Luke's House, London, 1894.

25. BARRINGTON, M. R., *****Report on Conference on Euthanasia, 19 December 1973, Royal Society of Health, London.

26. BEARD, P., 'Carcinoma of the Ovary', *N.T.*, 1978 (26 January), p. 140. (See also refs. 266, 308, 323, 424, 431.)

27. BENTLEY, G. B., Appendix 3 in 'Decisions About Life and Death', 1965 – booklet from Church Information Office, London. (See ref. 273.)

28. BIRLEY, M. F., *****'Terminal Care', *Almoner*, 1960, **13**, p. 86.

29. BIRTCHNELL, J., *****'Case Register Study of Bereavement', *P.R.S.M.*, 1970, **64**, p. 279. (See also refs. 30, 52.)

30. BIRTCHNELL, J., *****'Early Parent Death and Psychiatric Diagnosis', *Social Psychiatry*, 1972, **7**, p. 202.

31. BLACK, D., ******'Bereavement in Children', paper from 'Cruse'. (See also ref. 16.)

32. BLACK, D., ******'Working with Widowed Mothers', *Social Work Today*, 1976, **6**, p. 684. (See also ref. 31.)

33. BLACK, D., 'What Happens to Bereaved Children?', *P.R.S.M.*, 1976, **69**, p. 842.

34. BLACK, D., 'The Bereaved Child', *Journal of Child Psychology & Psychiatry*, 1978, **19**, p. 287.

35. BLAKE, P., 'Lying to the Dying', *W.M.*, 1977 (27 July), p. 32. (See also ref. 430.)

36. BLOOM, A. (Metropolitan Anthony), speech reported in Newsletter No. 20 (April 1972) of Institute of Religion & Medicine, St Margaret's Vicarage, St Margaret's Road, Oxford 2, England.

37. BONICA, J. J., 'Authorities and Teachers Neglect Cancer Pain Research', *Pain Topics*, 1978 (December), p. 1.

38. BOWLBY, J., *'Grief & Mourning in Infancy and Early Childhood', *Psychoanalytic Study of the Child*, 1960, **15**, p. 9. (See also ref. 40.)

39. BOWLBY, J., 'Processes of Mourning', *International Journal of Psychoanalysis*, 1961, **42**, p. 317.

40. BOWLBY, J., *'Pathological Mourning & Childhood Mourning', *Journal of the American Psychoanalysis Association*, 1963, **11**, p. 500.

41. BREWER, C., 'Murder Most Inefficient', *W.M.*, 1977 (19 October), p. 39; and 'Insufficient Evidence', *W.M.*, 1979 (13 January), p. 28. Reported in *Daily Telegraph*, London, 1979 (12 January), p. 9, 'No Prosecution Over Attempted Euthanasia'. (See also ref. 248.)

42. BRITISH JOURNAL OF GERIATRIC PRACTICE – editorial: 'An Alternative to Euthanasia', 1969 (March), p. 5. (See also refs. 62, 170, 176.)

43. BRITISH MEDICAL ASSOCIATION – booklet: 'The Problem of Euthanasia', January 1971, London. (See also ref. 393.)

44. B.M.J. – editorial: *'Termination of Life', 1971, **1**, p. 187. (See also ref. 61.)

45. B.M.J. – editorial: 'Treatment of Carcinoma of the Larynx', 1971, **1**, p. 417. (See also refs. 186, 197, 442.)

46. B.M.J. – editorial: 'Tragic Dilemma', 1972, **4**, p. 567.

47. B.M.J. – editorial: 'Unexpected Deaths of Babies', 1973, **1**, p. 308. (See also ref. 106.)

48. B.M.J. – editorial: 'Talking About Death', 1974, **2**, p. 131.

49. B.M.J. – editorial: 'Happy Death Day', 1975, **4**, p. 423.

50. B.M.J. – editorial: *'Pain and the Dissatisfied Dead', 1978, **1**, p. 459.

51. BROCKLEHURST, J. C., 'Co-ordination in the Care of the Elderly', *Lancet*, 1966, **1**, p. 1363. (See also ref. 408.)

52. BROWN, F., *'Depression & Childhood Bereavement', *Journal of Mental Science*, 1961, **107**, p. 754.

53. BROWN, F., *'Childhood Bereavement & Subsequent Psychiatric Disorder', *British Journal of Psychiatry*, 1966, **112**, p. 1035. (See also refs. 157, 407.)

54. CADE, S., 'Cancer: the Patient's Viewpoint and the Clinician's Problems', *P.R.S.M.*, 1963, **56**, p. 1. (See also refs. 208, 349.)

55. CAHILL, A., 'Cash Crisis Hits Scots Hospice', *Pulse*, 1978 (18 March), p. 10. (See also ref. 384.)

56. CALDWELL, J. R., 'The Management of Inoperable Malignant Disease in General Practice', *J.C.G.P.*, 1964, **8**, p. 23.

57. CALNAN, K., 'Details of Discharged Cancer Patients Sent to G.P.'s', *General Practitioner*, 1974 (11 October), p. 4.

58. CALVERT, P., et al., 'Death in a Country Area and Its Effect on the Health of Relatives', *Medical Journal of Australia*, 1977, **2**, p. 635. (See also refs. 132, 279, 433.)

59. CANG, S., 'Why Not a Hospital-At-Home Here?', *Age Concern Today*, 1976 (Winter), p. 9. (See also refs. 296, 398.)

60. CAVADINO & LAMERTON, *'Evidence to the Criminal Law Revision Committee re "Mercy Killing" Proposals', Human Rights Society, 27 Walpole Street, London SW3. (March 1977.)

61. CHRISTIE, M., 'Help at Hand', letter to *Hornsey Journal*, London, 1977 (4 March).

62. CLARK, A. N. G., 'Voluntary Euthanasia: Charlatan's Charter?', *W.M.*, 1977 (9 March), p. 71.

63. CLARK, A. N. G., 'The Practical Side of Choosing Death', letter to *Evening Argus*, Brighton, England, 1977 (31 August).

64. CLEMINSON, B., 'Management of Chronic Intractable Pain', letter to *Hospital Update*, 1976 (May), p. 261. (See also ref. 316.)

65. COPPERMAN, H., 'The Dying Need Company', letter to *N.M.*, 1976 (30 December), p. 32. (See also ref. 227.)

66. COPPERMAN, H., 'Foam-Stick Applicators', letter to *N.T.*, 1977 (31 March), p. 459.

67. COPPERMAN, H., 'Uncontrolled Pain Doesn't Justify Murder', letter to *Doctor*, 1978 (15 June). (See also ref. 309.)

68. COTTER, Z. M., *'Institutional Care of the Terminally Ill', *Hospital Progress*, 1971, **52**, p. 42.

69. COX, H., *The Church in the Secular City*, Penguin, London, 1968, p. 162.

70. CRAMOND, W. A., *'Psychotherapy of the Dying Patient', *B.M.J.*, 1970, **3**, p. 389.

71. CRAVEN & WALD, *'Hospice Care for Dying Patients', *A.J.N.*, 1975, **75**, p. 1816. (See also refs. 335, 389.)

72. CRONK, H. M., 'This Business of Dying', *N.T.*, 1972 (31 August), p. 1100. (See also ref. 210.)

73. CROOK, E., 'A Matter of Privacy', *N.M.*, 1977 (1 September), p. 28. (See also ref. 177.)

74. CURRAN, C., 'Is There a Right to Kill?', letter to *Sunday Telegraph*, London, 1969 (30 March).

75. CUSHING, H., *The Life of Sir William Osler*, Oxford University Press, 1940, **2**, p. 620 (1st edition 1925).

76. DAILY TELEGRAPH (London), 'Let Spina Bifidas Die, Says Doctor', 1972 (12 August). (See also ref. 365.)

77. DAILY TELEGRAPH – *editorial: 'Criminal Compassion', 1976 (29 September).

78. DANIEL, M. P., 'The Social Worker's Role', *B.M.J.*, 1973, **1**, p. 36.

79. DARROCH, J., 'How People Have Been Conned', letter to *The Scotsman*, Edinburgh, 1976 (22 October). (See also refs. 151, 366.)

80. DAUBE, D., 'Sanctity of Life', *P.R.S.M.*, 1967, **60**, p. 1235. (See also ref. 358.)

81. DAVIS, J. A., *'The Attitude of Parents to the Approaching Death of Their Child', *Developmental Medicine and Child Neurology*, 1964, **6**, p. 286. (See also refs. 352, 181.)

82. DAVISON, S., 'Diplomatosis Syndrome', letter to *N.M.*, 1977 (1 September), p. 12. (See also refs. 203, 294.)

83. DEUTSCH, H., *'Absence of Grief', *Psychoanalysis Quarterly*, 1937, **6**, p. 12.

84. DE VEBER, L. L., 'Terminally Ill Children', report in *C.M.A.J.*, 1978, **119**, p. 385. See: *University of Western Ontario Medical Journal*, 1977 (December), p. 18.

85. DOBIHAL, E. F., *'Talk or Terminal Care?', *Connecticut Medicine*, 1974, **38**, p. 364.

86. DONALDSON, M., 'Cancer, the Psychological Disease', *Lancet*, 1955, **1**, p. 959. (See also ref. 191.)

87. DOTT, N. M., 'Discussion on the Treatment of Intractable Pain', *P.R.S.M.*, 1959, **52**, p. 987.

88. DOWNIE, P. A., *'The Physiotherapist and the Patient with Cancer', *Physiotherapy*, 1971 (March), p. 117.

89. DOWNIE, P. A., 'Rehabilitation Following Mastectomy', *N.M.*, 1972 (15 September), p. 19. (See also ref. 90.)

90. DOWNIE, P. A., 'Persistent Cancer', *N.M.*, 1972 (29 September), p. 36.

91. DOWNING, A. B., 'Euthanasia and Christianity', reprint from *Modern Free Churchman*, Belfast, from Voluntary Euthanasia Society, London. (See also ref. 313.)

92. DOWNING, J. W., et al., 'Buprenorphine (Temgesic): Comparison with Morphine', *British Journal of Anaesthesia*, 1977, **49**, p. 251. (See also ref. 166.)

93. DOYLE, D., 'Dignity for Dying Patients', letter to *The Scotsman*, Edinburgh, 1978 (6 February).

94. DRINKWATER & ROBERTS, **'Cure or Care in Everyday Practice', *J.M.E.*, 1978, **4**, p. 12.

95. DRUG & THERAPEUTICS BULLETIN, 'Corticosteroids in Terminal Cancer', 1974, **12**, p. 63. (See also refs. 374, 400.)

96. DUBERLEY, J., 'The Clinical Nurse Specialist', *N.T.*, 1976 (18 November), p. 1794.

97. DUNEA, G., 'Death With Dignity', *B.M.J.*, 1976, **1**, p. 824.

98. DUNNET, S., 'I Know I Am Dying', *Sunday Times*, London (magazine section), 1973 (25 November). (See also ref. 148.)

99. DUNPHY, J. E., **'On Caring For the Patient with Cancer', *New England Journal of Medicine*, 1976, **295**, p. 313. (See also ref. 337.)

100. DUNSTAN, G. R., *'Mercy Killing: Does the Law Really Need to

Create a New Offence?', *The Times*, 1976 (30 November). (See also ref. 371.)

101. EARENGAY, W. G., 'Voluntary Euthanasia', *Medico-Legal Criminology Review*, 1940, **8**, p. 91.

102. EDWARDS & THOMPSON, 'Who Are the Fatherless?', *New Society*, London, 1971 (4 February), p. 192.

103. EDWARDS, L., 'I Killed for Love', *Woman's Own* (London), 1977 (17 May), p. 20.

104. ELLISON-NASH, D. F., 'Spina Bifida and Allied Disorders', *Hospital Medicine*, 1968, **2**, p. 439. (See also ref. 105.)

105. ELLISON-NASH, D. F., 'The Impact of Total Care, with Special Reference to Myelodysplasia', *Developmental Medicine and Child Neurology*, Supplement 22, 1970, p. 1.

106. EMERY, J. L., 'Welfare of Families of Children Found Unexpectedly Dead', *B.M.J.*, 1972, **1**, p. 612.

107. EMRYS-ROBERTS, R. M., 'Death and Resuscitation', letter to *B.M.J.*, 1969, **4**, p. 364.

108. ENGEL, G. L., *'Psychogenic Pain and the Pain-Prone Patient', *American Journal of Medicine*, 1959, **26**, p. 899.

109. EPICTETUS, *Dissertations* I, IX: 16. (See also ref. 301.)

110. EVANS, B., 'The Dying Child', *W.M.*, 1976 (24 March), p. 17.

111. EXTON-SMITH, A. N., *'Terminal Illness in the Aged', *Lancet*, 1961, **2**, p. 305. (See also refs. 158, 330.)

112. FAWELL, R. M., *Death is a Horizon*, booklet from Quaker Bookstall, Friends' House, Euston Road, London NW1. (See also ref. 327.)

113. FEIFEL, H., *'Perception of Death', *Annals of New York Academy of Sciences*, 1969, **164**, p. 669.
FEIFEL, H., 'Attitudes Toward Death – a Psychological Perspective', *Journal of Consulting and Clinical Psychology*, 1969, **33**, p. 292.

114. FIDLER, M., 'Prophylactic Internal Fixation of Secondary Neoplastic Deposits in Long Bones', *B.M.J.*, 1973, **1**, p. 341. (See also refs. 289, 292.)

115. FINLAY, H. V. L., 'Selecting Cases of Myelomeningocele for Surgery', *B.M.J.*, 1971, **3**, p. 429. (See also refs. 221, 223.)

116. FISHER, R. E. W., *'Death Penalty', letter to the *Lancet*, 1970, **1**, p. 299.

117. FLEW & TWYCROSS, *'Active and Passive Euthanasia', letter to *J.M.E.*, 1975, **1**, p. 153. (See also ref. 185.)

118. FLOOD, P., 'Morals and Medicine', booklet from Catholic Truth Society, London.

119. FORD & PINCHERLE, *'Arrangements for Terminal Care in the N.H.S.', *Health Trends*, 1978, **10**, p. 73. (See also ref. 353.)

120. FOX, T. F., 'The Greater Medical Profession', *Lancet*, 1956, **2**, p. 779.

121. FRASER, M., 'How to Recognise Pathological Grief Reactions', *Modern Geriatrics*, 1978 (May), p. 30.

122. FRETWELL, J. E., 'A Child Dies', *N.T.*, 1973 (5 July), p. 867. (See also ref. 138.)

123. GARDHAM, J., 'Palliative Surgery', *P.R.S.M.*, 1955, **48**, p. 703.

124. GARDNER & MYERSCOUGH, 'A New Approach to Abortion and Its Implications for the Euthanasia Debate', *J.M.E.*, 1975, **1**, pp. 127 and 130. (See also ref. 366.)

125. GARNER, J., 'Palliative Care: It's the Quality of Life Remaining that Matters', *C.M.A.J.*, 1976, **115**, p. 179. (See also ref. 260.)

126. GERLE, B., et al., *'The Patient with Inoperable Cancer from the Psychiatric and Social Standpoints', *Cancer*, 1960, **13**, p. 1206. (See also refs. 217, 429.)

127. GIBSON, R., 'Ethics & Management of Advanced Cancer', *B.M.J.*, 1962, **2**, p. 977. (See also ref. 270.)

128. GILES, L., *Musings of a Chinese Mystic*, Murray, London, 1955, p. 32.

129. GILLIE, O., 'Doctor Tells: Why I Killed 15 Patients', *Sunday Times*, London, 1974 (10 November). (See also refs. 155, 264, 351.)

130. GILLON, R., 'Voluntary Euthanasia', *Oxford Medical School Gazette*, 1964, **16**, p. 49. (See also ref. 372.)

131. GLICK, J. H., 'A Doctor's Prescription for Mercy', *Good Housekeeping*, New York, 1975, **181** (August), p. 67.

132. GOLDIE, L., *'Reactions to Death and Dying', paper from 'Cruse'. (See ref. 16.)

133. GOULD, D., 'A Better Way to Die', *New Statesman*, London, 1969 (4 April), p. 474.

134. GOULD, D., 'Some Lives Cost Too Dear', *New Statesman*, London, 1975 (21 November), p. 633. (See also ref. 192.)

135. GREEN, M., 'Care of the Child with a Long-Term Life-Threatening Illness', *Pediatrics*, 1967, **39**, p. 441.

136. GREER, G., 'Not a Time To Die', *Sunday Times*, London, 1972 (3 December).

137. GUSTERSON, F. R., *'Personal View', *B.M.J.*, 1975, **4**, p. 576.

138. GYULAY, J., *'Care of the Dying Child', *Nursing Clinics of North America*, 1976, **11**, p. 95.

139. HACKLEY, J. A., 'Affiliate of Nursing Home Group Develops Comprehensive Hospice Program in Tucson', *Hospitals* (Journal of American Hospitals Assoc.), 1977, **51**, p. 84. (See also ref. 370.)

140. HANCOCK, S., *'A Death in the Family: A Lay View', *B.M.J.*, 1973, **1**, p. 29.

141. HANSARD – HOUSE OF COMMONS, 1970 (7 April), **799**, pp. 252–8. (Also 21 February 1973, 3476 Notices of Questions & Motions No. 62 Mr Iremonger.)

142. HANSARD – HOUSE OF LORDS, *1936 (1st December), **103**, pp. 465–506.

143. HANSARD – HOUSE OF LORDS, *1950 (28 November), **169**, pp. 552–98.

144. HANSARD – HOUSE OF LORDS, **1969 (25 March), **300**, pp. 1143–1254. (See also ref. 390.)

145. HANSARD – HOUSE OF LORDS, **1976 (12 February), **368**, pp. 196–301.

146. HANSARD – HOUSE OF LORDS, 1976 (16 July), debate on 'The Family in Britain Today'.

147. HARDY, S. J., 'Caring for Children in Hospital'. Project Paper No. 4 from King's Fund Centre, 24 Nutford Place, London W1 (February 1974).

148. HARRIS, J., 'Living With Cancer', *Pulse*, 1974 (12 January), p. 19.

149. HARRISON, M. J. G., 'The Diagnosis of Brain Death', *British Journal of Hospital Medicine*, 1976 (October), p. 320. (See also ref. 222.)

150. HART, F. D., et al., *'Pain at Night', *Lancet*, 1970, **1**, p. 881.

151. HASKARD, O., *'Slippery Slope', letter to *The Times*, 1969 (29 March).

152. HASSETT, P., 'No Substitute for Love and Trust', *N.M.*, 1978 (28 September), p. 39. (See also ref. 236.)

153. HEENAN, J. C., 'The Need for Plain Speaking', letter to *The Times*, 1969 (26 March).

154. HELENA MARIE, SR., et al., *'Unnecessary Suffering', letter to *N.T.*, 1977 (3 February), p. 162. (See also refs. 256, 386.)

155. HENDERSON-SMITH, S. L., 'Death Fixation', letter to *Pulse*, 1973 (28 July), p.11. Answered by Lamerton, R., 'Hooray for the Statement', letter to *Pulse*, 1973 (18 August), p. 11.

156. HENKE, E., **Unpublished essay by a patient from St Christopher's Hospice, Lawrie Park Road, London SE26.

157. HILL & PRICE, *'Childhood Bereavement and Adult Depression', *British Journal of Psychiatry*, 1967, **113**, p. 743.

158. HINTON, J. M., **'The Physical and Mental Distress of the Dying', *Quarterly Journal of Medicine*, 1963, **32**, p.1.

159. HINTON, J. M., *'Facing Death', *Journal of Psychosomatic Research*, 1966, **10**, p. 22.

160. HINTON, J. M., *'Talking with People About to Die', *B.M.J.*, 1974, **3**, p. 25.

161. HOBSON, J. M., *Some Early and Later Houses of Pity*, George Routledge, London, 1926, pp. 1–3.

162. HOFFMAN, E., 'Don't Give Up On Me!', *A.J.N.*, 1971, **71**, p. 60. (See also ref. 198.)

163. HOLDEN, C., 'Hospices for the Dying: Relief from Pain and Fear', *Science*, 1976 (30 July), p. 389.

164. HOLFORD, J. M., 'Terminal Care', *N.T.* booklet, February 1973.

165. HORNS, W. H., et al., *'Plasma Levels and Symptom Complaints in Patients Maintained on Daily Dosage of Methadone Hydrochloride', *Clinical Pharmacology and Therapeutics*, 1975, **17**, p. 636. (See also refs. 174, 215, 382.)

166. HOVELL, B. C., *'Comparison of Buprenorphine (Temgesic), Pethidine and Pentazocine (Fortral) for Relief of Pain After Operation', *British Journal of Anaesthesia*, 1977, **49**, p. 913. (See also ref. 317.)

167. HOWARTH, R. V., *'The Psychiatry of Terminal Illness in Children', *P.R.S.M.*, 1972, **65**, p. 1039.

168. HOWELL, D., *'A Child Dies', *Journal of Pediatric Surgery*, 1966, **1**, p. 2.

169. HOY, A. M., 'Terminal Pain', *N.M.*, 1977 (10 March), p. 60. (See also refs. 385, 437.)

170. HUDSON-EVANS, R., **'Quality of Life', letter to *B.M.J.*, 1976, **3**, p. 48.

171. HUMAN RIGHTS SOCIETY, *'The Hospice Movement', leaflet, 1978. (See refs. 60, 340, 445.)

172. HUNT, J. M., et al., **'Patients with Protracted Pain: A Survey Conducted at the London Hospital', *J.M.E.*, 1977, **3**, p. 61.

173. INCURABLE PATIENTS BILL (House of Lords), 4 December 1975, H.M. Stationery Office.

174. INTURISSI & VEREBELY, 'Levels of Methadone in the Plasma in Methadone Maintenance', *Clinical Pharmacology and Therapeutics*, 1972, **13**, p. 633.

175. IRVINE & SMITH, *'Patterns of Visiting', *Lancet*, 1963, **1**, p. 597. (See also ref. 354.)

176. IRVINE, R. E., *'Progressive Patient Care in the Geriatric Unit', *Postgraduate Medical Journal*, 1963, **39**, p. 401.

177. ISAACS, B., 'May I Leave the Room, Nurse?', *N.M.*, 1978 (23 November), p. 24.

178. JANIS, I. L., *Psychological Stress: Psychoanalytic and Behavioural Studies of Surgical Patients*, Chapman & Hall, London, 1958. (See also refs. 228, 285.)

179. JESSOP, J., 'Their Death in Our Hands', *W.M.*, 1978 (12 July), p. 81.

180. JOLIN, C., 'Death Struggle Still Life?' *Pulse*, 1965 (13 February), p. 1.

181. JOLLY, H., 'What Your Child Wants to Know About Death', *The Times*, 1973 (3 October).

182. J.A.M.A. *'A Definition of Irreversible Coma – Report of the Ad Hoc Committee of Harvard Medical School to Examine the Definition of Brain Death', 1968, **205**, p. 337. (See also refs. 183, 184, 304, 343.)

183. J.A.M.A., 'Refinements in Criteria for the Determination of Death – An Appraisal', report from the Institute of Society, Ethics and Life Sciences, 1972, **221**, p. 48.

184. J.A.M.A. – *editorial: 'Harvard Criteria – An Appraisal', 1972, **221**, p. 65.

185. J.M.E. – editorial: 'Euthanasia', 1975, **1**, p. 1.

186. J.M.E. – *editorial: 'The Cost of Saving Life'; and Case Conference: 'Does the End Result Justify the Expense?', 1975, **1**, pp. 161 and 187.

187. J.M.E. – Case Conference: 'Retreat from Death', 1976, **2**, p. 200. (See also ref. 427.)

188. J.M.E. – *Case Conference: 'Strive Officiously to Keep Alive?', 1977, **3**, p. 189. (See also ref. 368.)

189. KASTENBAUM, R., *'Death and Responsibility', *Psychiatric Opinion*, 1966, **3**, pp. 5 and 35.

190. KAY, W. W., 'The Right to Die', letter to *The Times*, 1970 (1 May).
191. KELLY & FRIESEN, 'Do Cancer Patients Want to Be Told?', *Surgery*, 1950, **27**, p. 822.
192. KENNEDY, I. M., 'The Karen Quinlan Case: Problems and Proposals', *J.M.E.*, 1976, **2**, p. 3.
193. KENNEDY, I. M., 'The Legal Effect of Requests by the Terminally Ill and Aged Not to Receive Further Treatment from Doctors', *Criminal Law Review*, 1976 (April), p. 217.
194. KEYSER, M., *'At Home With Death: A Natural Child-Death', *Journal of Pediatrics*, 1977, **90**, p. 486.
195. KIRK, J., 'Cancer and the Patient', letter to *B.M.J.*, 1973, **4**, p. 164.
196. KOHN, J., 'Hospice Building Speaks on Many Emotional Levels to Patient, Family', *Modern Healthcare* – Short-term Care Edition, 1976, **5**, p. 56.
     KRON, J., *'Designing a Better Place to Die', *New York Magazine*, 1976 (1 March), p. 43.
197. KUBIK & DAS GUPTA, 'Survival After 195 Defibrillations', *B.M.J.*, 1969, **4**, p. 432.
198. KÜBLER-ROSS, E., 'What Is It Like to Be Dying?', *A.J.N.*, 1971, **71**, p. 54.
199. KÜBLER-ROSS & GOLEMAN, *'The Child Will Always Be There – Real Love Doesn't Die', *Psychology Today*, 1976 (September), pp. 44 and 48.
200. LAMERTON, E. W., 'Light and Darkness', p. 22 of *'Why Am I? What Am I? Who Am I?'*, Vantage Press, 516 West 34th Street, New York 10001 (1976).
201. LAMERTON, R., *'What Does Euthanasia Mean?', 1973, booklet from Church Literature Association, Faith House, Tufton Street, London SW1. (See also ref. 378.)
202. LAMERTON, R., 'Resurrected by an Enema', *N.T.*, 1976 (21 October), p. 1653.
203. LAMERTON, R., 'Care of the Dying – A Specialty', *N.T.*, 1978 (16 March), p. 436.
204. LANCET – editorial: *'Prolongation of Dying', 1962, **2**, p. 1205. (See also ref. 410.)
205. LANCET – editorial: 'Care of the Dying', 1965, **1**, p. 424.
206. LANCET – editorial: *'Limitations of Resuscitation', 1972, **1**, p. 1169.
207. LANCET – editorial: 'The Blocked Bed', 1972, **2**, p. 221.
208. LANCET – editorial: 'Operating On the Elderly', 1972, **2**, p. 489.
209. LANCET, 'Ethics of Selective Treatment of Spina Bifida: Report of the Bishop of Durham's Working Party', 1975, **1**, p. 85. (See also ref. 435.)
210. LANCET – editorial: *'Hospice Care', 1978, **1**, p. 1193.
211. LAPPÉ, M., *'Dying While Living: a Critique of Allowing-to-Die Legislation', *J.M.E.*, 1978, **4**, p. 195.
212. LESHAN & GASSMANN, *'Some Observations on Psychotherapy

with Patients Suffering from Neoplastic Diseases', *American Journal of Psychotherapy*, 1958, **12**, p. 723.

213. LESHAN, L. L., 'Psychological States as Factors in the Development of Malignant Disease', *Journal of the National Cancer Institutes*, 1959, **22**, p. 1.

214. LESHAN, L. L., ******'The World of the Patient in Severe Pain of Long Duration', *Journal of Chronic Diseases*, 1964, **17**, p. 119.

215. LESLIE, S. T., et al., 'Methadone: Evidence of Accumulation', letters to *B.M.J.*, 1977, **1**, pp. 375 and 1284.

216. LEVY & SCLARE, 'Fatal Illness in General Practice', *J.R.C.G.P.*, 1976, **26**, p. 303.

217. LEWIS, E., 'Cancer and the Patient', letter to *B.M.J.*, 1973, **4**, p. 164.

218. LIEGNER, L. M., 'St Christopher's Hospice, 1974', *J.A.M.A.*, 1975, **234**, p. 1047.

219. LINDEMANN, E., ******'Symptomatology and Management of Acute Grief', *American Journal of Psychiatry*, 1944, **101**, p. 141.

220. LIPMAN, A. G., ******'Drug Therapy in Terminally-Ill Patients', *American Journal of Hospital Pharmacy*, 1975, **32**, p. 270. (See also ref. 246.)

221. LLOYD-ROBERTS, G. C., 'Developments in Orthopaedic Surgery in Childhood', *N.M.*, 1972 (8 August), p. 33. (See also refs. 115, 223.)

222. LONGLEY, C., 'Wrong to Prolong Life at Any Cost, Dr Coggan Says', *The Times*, 1976 (14 December). See also the article 'The Last Taboo' in the same edition.

223. LORBER, J., 'Results of Treatment of Myelomeningocele', *Developmental Medicine and Child Neurology*, 1971, **13**, p. 279.

224. LYONS, R., 'Controlling the Symptons of Terminal Cancer', *Pulse*, 1979 (12 May), p. 40. (See also ref. 442.)

225. MACAULAY, T. B., *History of England*, 1849, **1**, p. 437.

226. MACDONALD, E. A., 'Cancer and the Patient', letter to *B.M.J.*, 1973, **4**, p. 492.

227. MACMILLAN, S., ******'Margaret – A Study in Perception', *N.T.*, 1972 (28 December), p. 1644.

228. MADDISON & WALKER, 'Factors Affecting the Outcome of Conjugal Bereavement', *British Journal of Psychiatry*, 1967, **113**, p. 1057.

229. MAGRAW, R. M., 'Grief – Its Clinical Importance and Its Resolution', *Modern Medicine*, 1973 (October), p. 554.

230. MARIE CURIE MEMORIAL FOUNDATION with the Queen's Institute of District Nursing. *****Report on a National Survey Concerning Patients with Cancer Nursed at Home. April 1952.

231. MARKS & SACHAR, 'Undertreatment of Medical Inpatients with Narcotic Analgesics', *Annals of Internal Medicine*, 1973, **78**, p. 173.

232. MASTERMAN, J., 'How the Right to Die Could Improve the Quality of Life', *The Times*, 1976 (20 October). (See also refs. 420, 440.)

233. MATT: 19. v. 17–18.
    EXODUS: 23. v. 7.

BUDDHAGHOSA – Papancasudani: Sutta 9 'The Five Precepts of the Buddha'.

234. MCCARTHY, D. G., 'The Use and Abuse of Cardiopulmonary Resuscitation', *Hospital Progress*, 1975 (April), **56**, p. 64.

235. MCCARTHY, D. G., 'Should Catholic Hospitals Sponsor Hospices?', *Hospital Progress*, 1976 (December), **57**, p. 61.

236. MCCLINTOCK, E. M., 'A Patient with Carcinomatosis Nursed At Home', *N.T.*, 1977 (24 March), p. 412.

237. MCNULTY, B. J., **'Discharge of the Terminally-Ill Patient', *N.T.*, 1970 (10 September), p. 1160.

238. MCNULTY, B. J., 'St. Christopher's Outpatients', *A.J.N.*, 1971, **71**, p. 2328.

239. MCNULTY, B. J., *'Continuity of Care', *B.M.J.*, 1973, **1**, p. 38.

240. MCNULTY, B. J., **'Domiciliary Care of the Dying: Some Problems Encountered', *N.M.*, 1973 (18 May), p. 29. (See also ref. 369.)

241. MCNULTY, B. J., 'Terminal Care in the Home', *Medical Digest*, 1973, **18**, p. 14.

242. MCNULTY, B. J., **'The Problem of Pain in the Dying Patient', *Queen's Nursing Journal*, 1973, **16**, p. 152.

243. MCNULTY, B. J., **'The Nurse's Contribution in Terminal Care', *N.M.*, 1974 (10 October), p. 59.

244. MCNULTY, B. J., *'Longevity and Loss', *N.T.*, 1977 (15 December), p. 1967. (See also ref. 341.)

245. MEISSNER, J. P., *'Euthanasia: A Legal Analysis of "Death-With-Dignity" Legislation', *Marriage and Family Newsletter*, 1978, **9**, p. 2 (P.O. Box 922, Peterborough, Ontario, Canada).

246. MELZACK, R., et al., **'The Brompton Mixture: Effects on Pain in Cancer Patients', *C.M.A.J.*, 1976, **115**, p. 125.

247. MILLARD, C. K., *'The Legalization of Voluntary Euthanasia', *Public Health*, 1931 (November), p. 39.

248. MILLARD, M., Thames Television 'Jimmy Young Show', 11 June 1974. Watered-down version is Case History A, p. 1. of 'On Dying Well' (see ref. 273).

249. MILLER & GWYNNE, 'Dependence, Independence and Counterdependence in Residential Institutions for Incurables', paper from Tavistock Institute of Human Relations, Belsize Lane, London NW3.

250. MILLER, M. B., 'Decision-Making in the Death Process of the Ill Aged', *Geriatrics*, 1971 (May), p. 105.

251. MILTON, G. W., *'The Care of the Dying', *Medical Journal of Australia*, 1972, **2**, p. 177. (See also ref. 284.)

252. MILTON, G. W., *'Thoughts in Mind of a Person with Cancer', *B.M.J.*, 1973, **4**, p. 221. (See also ref. 326.)

253. MOORE, A. R., 'Personal View', *B.M.J.*, 1978, **4**, p. 1363.

254. MOORE, E. G., Appendix 2 in 'Decisions About Life & Death', 1965, booklet from Church Information Office. (See ref. 273.)

255. MOORE, E. G., 'Doctor's Duty and Patient's Secrets', letter to *The Times*, 1971 (9 March).

256. MOORE, H., 'Nine Months in the Life of a Cancer Patient', *N.T.*, 1977 (13 January), p. 59.

257. MORETON, V., **'At St. Christopher's Hospice', *Physiotherapy*, 1969 (June), p. 68.

258. MOUNT, B. M., 'Death – A Part of Life', *Crux*, 1973–4, **11** (No. 3), p. 3 (745 Mount Pleasant Road, Toronto, Ontario, Canada).

259. MOUNT, B. M., et al., 'Death and Dying: Attitudes in a Teaching Hospital', *Urology*, 1974, **4**, p. 741. (See also ref. 387.)

260. MOUNT, B. M., **'The Problem of Caring for the Dying in a General Hospital: the Palliative Care Unit as a Possible Solution', *C.M.A.J.*, 1976, **115**, p. 119.

261. NAGY, M., **'The Child's Theories Concerning Death', *Journal of Genetic Psychology*, 1948, **73**, p. 3.

262. NATIONAL FEDERATION OF OLD AGE PENSIONS ASSOCIATIONS (91 Preston New Road, Blackburn, Lancs., England), Report of Conference at Douglas, 2–4 May 1972. Emergency Resolution 3, carried unanimously. (See also ref. 364.)

263. NATTERSON & KNUDSON, *'Observations Concerning the Fear of Death in Fatally Ill Children and Their Mothers', *Psychosomatic Medicine*, 1960, **22**, p. 456.

264. NEW YORK TIMES, American Euthanasia Society report, 1939 (27 January), p. 21, col. 7.

265. NICHOLSON, R., *'Should the Patient be Allowed to Die?', *J.M.E.*, 1975, **1**, p. 5.

266. NORTON, C., letters to *N.T.*, 1978: *'Nursing the Dying' (16 February), p. 273. *'Ways of Dying' (16 March), p. 461.

267. NORTON, J., 'Bedside Angels Are in Demand', *Pulse*, 1977 (23 April), p. 15.

268. N.T., 'Problems of Conscience: Quandary 3', 1976 (23 December), p. 2000. (See also refs. 290, 291, 369.)

269. N.T., Occasional Paper Supplement – 'Jewish Teaching Concerning Death', 1978 (23 March), p. 35.

270. N.T., Occasional Paper Supplement – 'Christian Teaching Concerning Death', 1978 (25 May), p. 58.

271. OGILVIE, H., *'Journey's End', *Practitioner*, 1957, **179**, p. 584.

272. OLSEN, G. D., 'Morphine Binding to Human Plasma Proteins', *Clinical Pharmacology and Therapeutics*, 1975, **17**, p. 31.

273. ON DYING WELL, *booklet from Church Information Office, 1974 (Church House, Dean's Yard, London SW1).

274. PAGE, I. H., 'Death and the Practitioner', editorial in *Modern Medicine*, 1970 (July), p. 605. (See also ref. 393.)

275. PAIN TOPICS, 'Study Throws Light on Who Put the Alcohol in a Brompton Cocktail', 1978 (October), p. 8. (See also ref. 383.)

276. PALLISTER, D., *'Daughter in Suicide Plot Gaoled for 2 Years', *Guardian*, London, 1977 (11 February).

277. PARKES, C. M., *'Recent Bereavement as a Cause of Mental Illness', *British Journal of Psychiatry*, 1964, **165**, p. 255. (See also ref. 314.)

278. PARKES, C. M., *'Bereavement and Mental Illness', *British Journal of Medical Psychology*, 1965, **38**, p. 1.

279. PARKES, C. M., **'Broken Heart', *B.M.J.*, 1969, **1**, p. 740.

280. PARKES, C. M., **'The First Year of Bereavement', *Psychiatry*, 1970, **33**, p. 444.

281. PARKES, C. M., **'Psychosocial Transitions', *Social Science and Medicine*, 1971, **5**, p. 101. (See also ref. 282.)

282. PARKES, C. M., *'Feelings of Mutilation and Grief Following Loss of a Limb, Spouse or Home', Lecture to the Society for Psychosomatic Research, London, 1 October 1971.

283. PARKES, C. M., *'Accuracy of Predictions of Survival in Later Stages of Cancer', *B.M.J.*, 1972, **2**, p. 29.

284. PARKES, C. M., 'The Patient's Right to Know the Truth', *P.R.S.M.*, 1973, **66**, p. 537.

285. PARKES, C. M., 'Unexpected and Untimely Bereavement: A Statistical Study of Young Boston Widows and Widowers'. A chapter in *Bereavement – Its Psychosocial Aspects* (p. 119), ed. Schoenberg, B., et al., Columbia University Press, New York, 1975.

286. PARKES, C. M., 'The Emotional Impact of Cancer of Ear, Nose and Throat on Patients and Their Families', *Journal of Laryngology and Otology*, 1975, **89**, p. 1271.

287. PARKES, C. M., **'Determinants of Outcome Following Bereavement', *Omega*, 1975, p. 303.

288. PARKES, C. M., **'Home or Hospital? Terminal Care as Seen by Surviving Spouses', *J.R.C.G.P.*, 1978, **28**, p. 19.

289. PARRISH & MURRAY, 'Surgical Treatment for Secondary Neoplastic Fractures', *Journal of Bone and Joint Surgery*, 1970, **52A**, p. 665.

290. PATON, A., 'Personal View', *B.M.J.*, 1969, **3**, p. 591.

291. PELLS, J., 'Pressures of Progress', *N.T.*, 1974 (21 February), p. 258.

292. PENN, C. R. H., 'Single Dose and Fractionated Palliative Irradiation for Osseous Metastases', *Clinical Radiology*, 1976, **27**, p. 405.

293. PERKINS, G., 'Resuscitation', letter to *Lancet*, 1967, **2**, p. 388. (See also ref. 428.)

294. PFEIFFER & LEMON, *'A Pilot Study in the Home Care of Terminal Cancer Patients', *American Journal of Public Health*, 1953, **43**, p. 909.

295. PICKERING, G., 'Medicine and Society', *B.M.J.*, 1971, **1**, p. 191.

296. PIGACHE, P., 'Who Goes Home?', *W.M.*, 1977 (30 November), p. 93.

297. PIUS XII, *'Concerning Re-animation'. Address to the International Congress of Anaesthetists, 24 February 1957. Translated in Catholic Truth Society booklet 'The Relief of Pain'.

298. PIUS XII, *Fatalities in Anaesthesia & Surgery – Answer to a question on 24 November 1957. Quoted by Vincent Collins, *J.A.M.A.*, 1960, **172**, p. 549.

299. PLATT, R., 'Reflections on Aging and Death', *Lancet*, 1963, **1**, p. 1. (See also ref. 363.)

300. PLAYER, A., ******'Casework in Terminal Illness', *Almoner*, 1954, **6**, p. 456.

301. PLINY, *Epistles*, I: 22.

302. POTTER, K., 'My Universe', *N.M.*, 1977 (17 November), p. 28.

303. PRENTICE, D., 'A Personal Story', *Quaker Monthly*, London, 1973 (October), p. 193.

304. PULSE, 'Drugs Complicate Brain Death Diagnosis', 1977 (14 May), p. 27.

305. RADFORD & WRIGHT, ***'Can Bereaved Relatives and Hospitals Help One Another?', *W.M.*, 1978 (22 February), p. 53.

306. REED, N., letters to *Daily Telegraph*, London, 1976: 'The Patient's Wish' (25 May); 'The Right to Die' (29 June). (See also ref. 347.)

307. REED, N., 'Voluntary Euthanasia', letter to *On Call*, 1977 (14 April), p. 15.

308. REED, N., 'Approaches to Death', letter to *N.T.*, 1978 (2 March), p. 372.

309. REED, N., ***'Poll Showed Public Backs Right to Die', letter to *Doctor*, 1978 (18 May).

310. REES, W. D., 'Personal View', *B.M.J.*, 1971, **2**, p. 164.

311. REES, W. D., ***'The Hallucinations of Widowhood', *B.M.J.*, 1971, **4**, p. 37.

312. REES, W. D., ***'Distress of the Dying', *B.M.J.*, 1972, **3**, p. 105.

313. REILLY, W. J., 'Personal View', *B.M.J.*, 1974, **3**, p. 465.

314. RICKARBY, G. A., 'Four Cases of Mania Associated with Bereavement', *Journal of Nervous and Mental Diseases*, 1977, **165**, p. 255.

315. RIDING, J. E., 'The Outpatient Pain Clinic', *Journal of the Royal College of Surgeons of Ireland*, 1966, **2**, p. 279.

316. ROBBIE, D. S., 'The Pain Clinic in a Cancer Hospital', *Excerpta Medica* International Conference Series, No. 200, 1968, p. 961.

317. ROBBIE & SAMARASINGHE, ***'Comparison of Aspirin-Codeine (Codis) and Paracetamol-Dextropropoxyphene (Distalgesic) Compound Tablets with Pentazocine (Fortral) for the Relief of Cancer Pain', *Journal of International Medical Research*, 1973, **1**, p. 246.

318. ROBINS, E., et al., 'Anticipatory Grief and Widowhood', *British Journal of Psychiatry*, 1973, **122**, p. 47.

319. RYDER & ROSS, 'Terminal Care – Issues & Alternatives', *Public Health Reports* (U.S.A.), 1977, **92**, p. 20.

320. ST CHRISTOPHER'S HOSPICE, Annual Reports (see ref. 156): ***1966–7, p. 24, 1977–8, p. 17.

321. ST. JOHN-STEVAS, N., 'Dying in Peace', letter to *The Times*, 1969 (25 March).

322. SAMPSON, W. I., ***'Dying At Home', *J.A.M.A.*, 1977, **238**, p. 2405.

323. SAUNDERS, B. M., et al., 'Approaches to Death', letter to *N.T.*, 1978 (2 March), p. 371.

324. SAUNDERS, B. M., 'Care of the Dying', letter to *N.T.*, 1978 (13 April), p. 637.

325. SAUNDERS, C. M., **'Treatment of Intractable Pain in Terminal Cancer', *P.R.S.M.*, 1963, **56**, p. 191.

326. SAUNDERS, C. M., **'Telling Patients', *District Nursing*, 1965, **8**, p. 149.

327. SAUNDERS, C. M., **'Watch With Me', *N.T.*, 1965 (26 November), p. 1615.

328. SAUNDERS, C. M., *'Death and Responsibility – A Medical Director's View', *Psychiatric Opinion*, 1966, **3**, pp. 3 and 35.

329. SAUNDERS, C. M., 'The Care of the Dying', *Gerontologia Clinica*, 1967, **9**, p. 6.

330. SAUNDERS, C. M., 'The Care of the Terminal Stages of Cancer', *Annals of the Royal College of Surgeons*, 1967, Supplement to Vol. **41**, p. 162.

331. SAUNDERS, C. M., *'St Christopher's Hospice', *British Hospital Journal and Social Service Review*, 1967 (10 November). Copies can be bought from St Christopher's Hospice (ref. 156), (See also ref. 419.)

332. SAUNDERS & WINNER, *'A Patient's Trust', letter to *The Times*, 1969 (27 March).

333. SAUNDERS, C. M., 'The Management of Fatal Illness in Childhood', *P.R.S.M.*, 1969, **62**, p. 550.

334. SAUNDERS, C. M., *'Training for the Practice of Clinical Gerontology: the Role of Social Medicine', *Interdisciplinary Topics in Gerontology*, 1970, **5**, p. 72.

335. SAUNDERS, C. M., **'The Need for In-Patient Care for the Patient with Terminal Cancer', *Middlesex Hospital Journal*, London, 1973 (February), p. 125.

336. SAUNDERS, C. M., *'Care for the Dying', *Patient Care* (Brussels), 1976, **3**, No. 6. Copies can be bought from St Christopher's Hospice (see ref. 156).

337. SAUNDERS, C. M., **'This House Believes Some Form of Voluntary Euthanasia Should Be Legalized', *W.M.*, 1978 (20 September), p. 45.

338. SEAL, P. V., 'A Fatal Case of Carcinoma in a Young Man', *J.C.G.P.*, 1965, **10**, p. 310.

339. SHEPHARD, D. A. E., 'Terminal Care – Towards an Ideal' (editorial), *C.M.A.J.*, 1976, **115**, p. 97.

340. SHEPHARD, D. A. E., *'Principles and Practice of Palliative Care', *C.M.A.J.*, 1977, **116**, p. 522.

341. SHINWELL, E., 'Old Age – A Time of Opportunity', pamphlet from Human Rights Society (see ref. 60), 1974.

342. SHOLIN, P. D., 'Death of a Son', *Woman's Own* (London), 1968 (10 December), p. 11.

343. SILVERMAN, D., et al., 'Cerebral Death and the Electroencephalogram', *J.A.M.A.*, 1969, **209**, p. 1505.

344. SIMPSON, M. A., *'If You Have Tiers, Prepare to Shed Them Now', *W.M.*, 1977 (4 May), p. 7. (See ref. 441.)

345. SKILLMAN, J. J., 'Ethical Dilemmas in the Care of the Critically Ill', *Lancet*, 1974, 2, p. 634.

346. SLATER, E. T. O., 'The Case for Voluntary Euthanasia', *Contemporary Review* (London), 1971, 219, No. 1267.

347. SLATER, E. T. O., 'Health Service or Sickness Service?', *B.M.J.*, 1971, 4, p. 734.

348. SMITH, T., 'This Honest Approach to Cancer', *The Times*, 1977 (20 December). (See also ref. 438.)

349. SMITHERS, D. W., *A Clinical Prospect of the Cancer Problem*, Livingstone, London, 1960, p. 150.

350. SMITHERS, D. W., *'Where to Die', *B.M.J.*, 1973, 1, p. 34. (See also ref. 415.)

351. SMOKER, B., *'Euthanasia', *Freethinker* (London) (March 1975). Letter to *The Times*, 1973 (22 January). Quoted in 'The Human Foetus', *Catholic Herald* (London), 1973 (13 July), by Bowman, P.

352. SOLNIT & GREEN, 'Psychologic Considerations in the Management of Deaths on Pediatric Hospital Services', *Pediatrics*, 1959, 24, p. 106.

353. SOUKOP & CALMAN, 'Cancer Patients: Where Do They Die?', *Practitioner*, 1977, 219, p. 838.

354. SPECK, P., *'The Hospital Visitor', *N.T.*, 1973 (5 July), p. 878.

355. SPINETTA, J. J., et al., 'Anxiety in the Dying Child', *Pediatrics*, 1973, 52, p. 841.

356. SPINKS, M. E., 'It *Has* Happened to Me', *N.T.*, 1970 (9 April), p. 461.

357. SPON, *Household Manual*, 1894, E. & F. N. Spon, London, 1st edn, 1887.

358. STARZL, T. E., 'Ethical Problems in Organ Transplantation', *Annals of Internal Medicine*, 1967, Supplement 7 to Vol. 67, p. 32.

359. SUICIDE ACT, 3 August 1961, Clause 2, H.M. Stationery Office.

360. SUTTON, M., 'Enlightened Attitude to Cancer', letter to *B.M.J.*, 1971, 2, p. 336.

361. SWEETINGHAM, C. R., *'Voluntary Euthanasia: Questions of Confidence', letter to *The Times*, 1969 (25 March). (See also ref. 392.)

362. TANNER, E. R., *'A Dedicated Nurse?', *N.T.*, 1962 (8 June), p. 221.

363. TANNER, E. R., 'The Postponement of Death in Old People', *Guy's Hospital Gazette*, London, 1972 (7 October), p. 511.

364. THOMSON, W., 'Aged Might Live in Fear of Euthanasia', *Daily Telegraph*, London, 1974 (19 November).

365. THE TIMES, *'Let These Children Die', correspondence throughout August 1972.

366. THE TIMES – editorial: *'The Taking of Life', 1970 (7 April).

367. THE TIMES – editorial: *'Too Merciful to Mercy Killers', 1976 (29 September).

368. TOWERS, B., *'The Impact of the California Natural Death Act', *J.M.E.*, 1978, 4, p. 96.

369. TOWNSEND, P., *The Last Refuge*, Routledge & Kegan Paul, London, 1962.

370. TRASKA, M. R., 'Hillhaven Negotiates for N.C.I. Grant', *Modern Healthcare*, 1977 (September), p. 40.

371. TUNKEL, V., 'Mercy Killing', letter to *The Times*, 1976 (4 October).

372. TWYCROSS, R. G., 'Euthanasia – An Alternative View', *Oxford Medical School Gazette*, 1964, 16, p. 103.

373. TWYCROSS, R. G., 'Principles and Practice of the Relief of Pain in Terminal Cancer', *Update*, 1972 (July). Copies can be bought from St Christopher's Hospice (see ref. 156).

374. TWYCROSS, R. G., 'How Steroids Can Help Terminal Cancer Patients', *General Practitioner*, 1972 (18 August), p. 13.

375. TWYCROSS & GILHOOLEY, *'Euphoriant Elixirs', letter to *B.M.J.*, 1973, 4, p. 552.

376. TWYCROSS, R. G., 'Clinical Experience with Diamorphine in Advanced Malignant Disease', *International Journal of Clinical Pharmacology, Therapy and Toxicology*, 1974, 9, p. 184.

377. TWYCROSS, R. G., *'The Use of Narcotic Analgesics in Terminal Illness', *J.M.E.*, 1975, 1, p. 10.

378. TWYCROSS, R. G., **'A Plea for Eu Thanatos', *The Month*, 1975 (February), p. 36. (114 Mount Street, London W1.)

379. TWYCROSS, R. G., *'Relief of Terminal Pain', *B.M.J.*, 1975, 4, p. 212.

380. TWYCROSS & WALD, *'Long Term Use of Diamorphine in Advanced Cancer', in Vol. 1 of *Advances in Pain Research and Therapy*, ed. J. J. Bonica, Raven Press, New York, 1976.

381. TWYCROSS, R. G., **'Choice of Strong Analgesic in Terminal Cancer: Diamorphine or Morphine?', *Pain*, 1977, 3, p. 93.

382. TWYCROSS, R. G., *'A Comparison of Diamorphine-with-Cocaine and Methadone', *British Journal of Clinical Pharmacology*, 1977, 4, p. 691.

383. TWYCROSS, R. G., *'Value of Cocaine in Opiate-Containing Elixirs', letter to *B.M.J.*, 1977, 4, p. 1348.

384. TWYCROSS, R. G., 'Patients "On Loan" from G.P.'s at Oxford's Continuing Care Unit', *Pain Topics*, 1977 (December), p. 4.

385. TWYCROSS, R. G., 'Recognising the Priorities for Effective Pain Control', *Pain Topics*, 1978 (October), p. 3.

386. TWYCROSS, R. G., **'Assessment of Pain in Advanced Cancer', *J.M.E.*, 1978, 4, p. 112.

387. VACHON, M. L. S., et al., *'The Final Illness in Cancer: the Widow's Perspective', *C.M.A.J.*, 1977, 117, p. 1151.

388. VERE, D. W., *'Should Christians Support Voluntary Euthanasia?', booklet from Christian Medical Fellowship (56 Kingsway, London WC2), 1971.

389. VERSPIEREN, P., 'Un Centre Anglais du Traitement de la Douleur', *Médecine De L'Homme* (Paris), 1975 (October), p. 10.

390. VOLUNTARY EUTHANASIA BILL (HL) BS 91/1 1968–9: 4.

391. VOLUNTARY EUTHANASIA SOCIETY (13 Prince of Wales Terrace, London W8), 'A Plea for Legislation to Permit Voluntary Euthanasia', booklet, 1970.

392. VOLUNTARY EUTHANASIA SOCIETY, *'Doctors and Euthanasia', booklet, 1971.

393. WALDRON & VICKERSTAFF, 'Necropsy Rates in the United Birmingham Hospitals', *B.M.J.*, 1975, **2**, p. 326.

394. WALLACE, L., 'The Needs of the Dying', *N.T.*, 1969 (13 November), p. 1450.

395. WARD, A. M. W., 'Telling the Patient', *J.R.C.G.P.*, 1974, **24**, p. 465. (See also ref. 422.)

396. WARD, A. M. W., 'Terminal Care in Malignant Disease', *Social Science and Medicine*, 1974, **8**, p. 413.

397. WARD, A. M. W., *'Terminal Care Homes', *Hospital and Health Services Review*, 1975 (July), p. 233.

398. WATKIN, B., 'Hospitals At Home', *N.M.*, 1978 (2 February), p. 10.

399. WATSON, L., 'Calcium Metabolism and Cancer', *Australian Annals of Medicine*, 1966, **15**, p. 359.

400. WATSON, L., *'Diagnosis and Treatment of Hypercalcaemia', *B.M.J.*, 1972, **2**, p. 150.

401. WATTS, G., 'Will the Tissue and the Rabbit Help the Addict?', *W.M.*, 1977 (16 November), p. 23.

402. WEATHERHEAD, L. D., *'Claiming the Right to Die', letter to *The Times*, 1970 (17 April).

403. WEISMAN & HACKETT, *'Predeliction to Death', *Psychosomatic Medicine*, 1961, **23**, p. 232.

404. WEISMAN & WORDEN, *'Psychosocial Analysis of Cancer Deaths', *Omega*, 1975, **6**, p. 61.

405. WELLDON, R. M. C., 'Living with Death', Part 56 of the *Book of Life – Marshall Cavendish Encyclopaedia*, 1969.

406. WELLDON, R. M. C., *'Bearing the Unbearable'. Part 97 of *Book of Life* (see ref. 405).

407. WELLDON, R. M. C., 'The Shadow of Death', *Family Process*, 1971, **10**, p. 281.

408. WEST, T. S., 'The G.P. and the Dying Patient', *Modern Geriatrics*, 1976 (November), p. 42.

409. WEST & HOLMES, 'Care of the Dying', *N.M.*, Nursing Care Supplement, 1977 (17 November).

410. WHITE, D., *'Death Control', *New Society*, London, 1972 (30 November), p. 502.

411. WHITEHEAD, T., 'Nurse or Doctor?', *W.M.*, 1976 (3 November), p.109.

412. WHITEHORN, K., *'We All Run Away, But Can't Escape', *Observer*, London (review section), 1968 (14 January).

413. WILKES, E., *'Cancer Outside Hospital', *Lancet*, 1964, **1**, p. 1379. (See also ref. 415.)

414. WILKES, E., *'Terminal Cancer at Home', *Lancet*, 1965, **1**, p. 799.

415. WILKES, E., *'Where to Die', *B.M.J.*, 1973, **1**, p. 32.

416. WILKES, E., *'Terminal Care and the Special Nursing Unit', *N.T.*, 1975 (9 January), p. 57. (See also ref. 417.)

417. WILKES, E., et al., 'A Different Kind of Day Hospital – For Patients with Preterminal Cancer and Chronic Disease', *B.M.J.*, 1978, **2**, p. 1053.

418. WILLIAMS, G., *'Euthanasia', *P.R.S.M.*, 1970, **63**, p. 663.

419. WILMERS, M., 'A Very Nice Place', *New Society*, London, 1974 (12 December), p. 669.

420. WILSHAW, C., 'The Right to Die', booklet from British Humanist Association (same address as Voluntary Euthanasia Society), 1974.

421. WILSON, F. G., 'Social Isolation and Bereavement', *Lancet*, 1970, **2**, p. 1356.

422. WILSON & FLETCHER, 'Communicating with the Dying', *J.M.E.*, 1975, **1**, p. 18.

423. WINNER, A. L., *'Death and Dying', *Journal of the Royal College of Physicians of London*, 1970, **4**, p. 351.

424. WITHERS, G., 'Approaches to Death', letter to *N.T.*, 1978 (2 March), p. 371.

425. WITZEL, L., *'Behaviour of the Dying Patient', *B.M.J.*, 1975, **2**, p. 81.

426. WOLVERHAMPTON EXPRESS & STAR (England), answer to 'Let These Children Die', 1972 (19 August).

427. WOODLEY, B., 'A Policy of Honesty', *Doctor*, 1974 (10 October), p. 9.

428. WOOTTON, B., 'The Right to Die', *New Society*, London, 1978 (26 October), p. 202.

429. WRIGHT, C., 'Personal View', *B.M.J.*, 1973, **4**, p. 45.

430. WRIGHT, J., 'The Unspoken Question', *Journal of Community Nursing*, 1978 (October), p. 4.

431. WRIGHT, P., 'Approaches to Death', letter to *N.T.*, 1978 (2 March), p. 371.

432. YALOM & GREAVES, 'Group Therapy with the Terminally Ill', *American Journal of Psychiatry*, 1977, **134**, p. 396.

433. YOUNG, M., et al., 'Mortality of Widowers', *Lancet*, 1963, **2**, p. 454.

434. YUDKIN, S., *'Children and Death', *Lancet*, 1967, **1**, p. 37. (See also ref. 194.)

435. ZACHARY & LORBER, *'Spina Bifida: To Treat or Not to Treat?', *N.M.*, 1978 (14 September), p. 13.

436. ZINSSER, H., *Spring, Summer and Autumn – Poems*, Alfred A. Knopf, New York, 1942.

437. ZORAB, J. S. M., 'It's the Normal Routine', *W.M.*, 1978 (28 June), p. 28.

438. ZORZA, V. & R., *'The Death of a Daughter', *Guardian*, London, 1978 (25 February), p. 9.

ADDENDA

439. KOHN, J., 'Hospice Movement Provides Human Alternative for Terminally Ill Patients', *Modern Healthcare*, Short Term Care Edition, 1976, **6**, p. 26.

440. SACKETT, W. W., 'Death with Dignity', *Medical Opinion and Review*, 1969, **5**, p. 25.

441. SIMPSON, M. A., *'Planning for Terminal Care', *Lancet*, 1976, **2**, p. 192.

442. HYAMS, D. E., 'Gastro-Intestinal Problems in the Old – Dysphagia', *B.M.J.*, 1974, **1**, p. 107.

443. LAMERTON, R., 'Cancer Patients Dying at Home', *Practitioner*, 1979, **223**, p. 813.

444. VEATCH, R., *Death, Dying and the Biological Revolution*, Chapter 4, pp. 116–63, Yale University Press, New Haven and London, 1976.

445. KASHIWAGI, T., *'The Organised Care of the Dying Patient', Proceedings of 4th Congress of the International College of Psychosomatic Medicine. From the author, Yodogawa Christian Hospital, Osaka, Japan.

446. KOOCHER, G. P., *'Talking With Children About Death', *American Journal of Orthopsychiatry*, 1974, **44**, p. 404.

447. ROSE & PORIES, 'Some Additional Notes on Hospice', *Ohio State Medical Journal*, 1977, **73**, p. 379. (See also refs. 85, 235.)

American Drug Names

Chemical name	Trade name: G.B.	Trade name: U.S.
Chlorpromazine	Largactil	Thorazine
Danthron and Poloxamer	Dorbanex	Peri-colase and Dorbantyl are similar
Disposable phosphate enema	Fletcher's enema	Fleet's enema
Methotrimeprazine	Veractil	Levoprome (U.S.) Nozinan (Canada)
Dextropropoxyphene	Distalgesic (with paracetamol)	Darvon
Prochlorperazine	Stemetil	Compazine
Pethidine	—	Demerol
Cylizine	Valoid	Marezine
Metoclopramide	Maxolon	Reglan

Index